Essentials of Clinical Microbiology

Essentials of Clinical Microbiology

M.S. Alam

Oxford Book Company
Jaipur ■ New Delhi

Published By

Oxford Book Company

Regd. Off. "Bony Residency", Gate No. 2
Opp. Tilak Public School, Vishweswariya Nagar,
Gopalpura Road, Jaipur - 302018, India
Ph: 0141 - 2761280, Telefax: 2761381
email - oxfordbookjpr@gmail.com
website - oxfordbookcompany.com

Delhi Office: 102, 1st Floor, Satyam House,
4327/3, Ansari Road, Darya Ganj,
New Delhi - 110002, India
Ph: 011-45652440

Distributed By
KEYA INTERNATIONAL PRESS LLP
E-mail: keyainternationalpressllp@gmail.com

First published in India, 2026

ISBN : 978-93-5524-245-7

Typeset by Shivangi Computers, Jaipur

Printed and bound in India by Thomson Press Ltd.,
New Delhi

Contents

Preface

The science of clinical microbiology is a dynamic interface where the microscopic world meets the macroscopic manifestations of disease. It is a field rooted in the understanding of invisible yet immensely powerful life forms that can both jeopardize and preserve human health. At its core, clinical microbiology delves into the identification, behaviour, and treatment implications of microorganisms responsible for infectious diseases—chief among them: bacteria, viruses, fungi, and parasites.

In this domain, the clinical microbiologist serves not merely as a diagnostician but as a sentinel of public health—decoding the nature of pathogens, tracing their transmission pathways, deciphering their adaptive strategies, and recommending precision-driven therapeutic solutions. Their expertise becomes vital in combating emergent resistance, curbing community outbreaks, and contributing to global strategies for epidemic and pandemic control. While a significant portion of their work revolves around harmful microbes, these specialists also investigate benign and beneficial microbial species to uncover novel avenues in antimicrobial development and immunotherapy.

The art of microbial detection has evolved into a sophisticated synergy of classical methodologies and modern molecular innovations. Biochemical assays continue to offer rapid insights through metabolic fingerprinting, enabling genus- and species-level identification. High-throughput platforms such as automated Vitek systems empower laboratories to conduct expansive diagnostic profiling with exceptional speed and accuracy. In parallel, serological techniques provide an elegant method to detect antigens and antibodies with extraordinary sensitivity—offering indispensable value in both bacterial and viral diagnostics.

Molecular biology has transformed the landscape further. Real-time PCR, with its capacity for simultaneous amplification and detection, has replaced time-intensive traditional protocols, eliminating the post-PCR risks of contamination and offering immediate clarity on microbial presence. This technique has revolutionized diagnostics for critical viral diseases, from HIV to Hepatitis, and forms the backbone of genomic comparisons between novel pathogens and established reference strains. Through these insights, clinicians and researchers can determine not only the origin of infection but also the optimal course of treatment, contributing to more informed and targeted medical care.

The relevance of this discipline extends far beyond the lab bench. Clinical microbiology empowers physicians, technologists, public health officials, and researchers with knowledge that directly influences patient outcomes and healthcare systems. From the hospital ward to the national health board, decisions grounded in microbiological evidence shape the future of disease management and prevention.

This book, Essentials of Clinical Microbiology, has been meticulously crafted to meet the intellectual and professional needs of those engaged in the field—from DMLT and M.Sc. students preparing for competitive examinations, to practicing lab technicians, pathology residents, medical students, and clinical consultants. It also serves as a reliable reference for MBBS faculty and science graduates seeking to embed microbiological principles within real-world clinical contexts. Supplemented with guided further readings and an updated compendium of antimicrobial agents in the appendix, this book stands as a practical, authoritative, and forward-looking resource in the ever-evolving arena of clinical microbiology.

— ***M.S. Alam***

Chapter

1

Factors Influencing Immunogenicity

Chemical Nature of Immunogens

The vast majority of immunogens are *proteins*. These may be pure proteins or they may be glycoproteins or lipoproteins. In general, proteins are usually very good immunogens.

Pure *polysaccharides* and lipopolysaccharides are good immunogens.

Nucleic acids are usually poorly immunogenic. However, they may become immunogenic when single stranded or when complexed with proteins.

In general *lipids* are non-immunogenic, although they may be haptens.

Types of Antigens

T-independent Antigens

T-independent antigens are antigens which can directly stimulate the B cells to produce antibody without the requirement for T cell help In general, polysaccharides are T-independent antigens.

The responses to these antigens differ from the responses to other antigens.

Properties of T-independent Antigens

1. Polymeric structure: These antigens are characterized by the same antigenic determinant repeated many times.
2. Polyclonal activation of B cells: Many of these antigens can activate B cell clones specific for other antigens (polyclonal activation). T-independent antigens can be subdivided into Type 1 and Type 2 based on their ability to polyclonally activate B cells. Type 1 T-independent antigens are polyclonal activators while Type 2 are not.
3. Resistance to degradation: T-independent antigens are generally more resistant to degradation and thus they persist for longer periods of time and continue to stimulate the immune system.

T-dependent Antigens

T-dependent antigens are those that do not directly stimulate the production of antibody without the help of T cells. Proteins are T-dependent antigens. Structurally these antigens are characterized by a few copies of many different antigenic determinants.

Hapten-carrier Conjugates

Hapten-carrier conjugates are immunogenic molecules to which haptens have been covalently attached. The immunogenic molecule is called the carrier.

Structure

Structurally these conjugates are characterized by having native antigenic determinants of the carrier as well as new determinants created by the hapten (haptenic determinants). The actual determinant created by the hapten consists of the hapten and a few of the adjacent residues, although the antibody produced to the determinant will also react with free hapten. In such conjugates the type of carrier determines whether the response will be T-independent or T-dependent.

Antigenic Determinants

Determinants Recognized by B Cells

1. Composition: Antigenic determinants recognized by B cells and the antibodies secreted by B cells are created by the primary sequence of residues in the polymer (linear or sequence

determinants) and/or by the secondary, tertiary or quaternary structure of the molecule (conformational determinants).

2. Size: In general antigenic determinants are small and are limited to approximately 4-8 residues. (amino acids and or sugars). The combining site of an antibody will accommodate an antigenic determinant of approximately 4-8 residues.
3. Number: Although, in theory, each 4-8 residues can constitute a separate antigenic determinant, in practice, the number of antigenic determinants per antigen is much lower than what would theoretically be possible. Usually the antigenic determinants are limited to those portions of the antigen that are accessible to antibodies.

Determinants Recognized by T Cells

1. Composition: Antigenic determinants recognized by T cells are created by the primary sequence of amino acids in proteins. T cells do not recognize polysaccharide or nucleic acid antigens. This is why polysaccharides are generally T-independent antigens and proteins are generally T-dependent antigens. The determinants need not be located on the exposed surface of the antigen since recognition of the determinant by T cells requires that the antigen be proteolytically degraded into smaller peptides. Free peptides are not recognized by T cells, rather the peptides associate with molecules coded for by the major histocompatibility complex (MHC) and it is the complex of MHC molecules + peptide that is recognized by T cells.
2. Size: In general antigenic determinants are small and are limited to approximately 8-15 amino acids.
3. Number: Although, in theory, each 8-15 residues can constitute a separate antigenic determinant, in practice, the number of antigenic determinants per antigen is much less than what would theoretically be possible. The antigenic determinants are limited to those portions of the antigen that can bind to MHC molecules. This is why there can by differences in the responses of different individuals.

Superantigens

When the immune system encounters a conventional T-dependent antigen, only a small fraction (1 in 10^4 -10^5) of the T cell population is able to recognize the antigen and become activated (monoclonal/

oligoclonal response). However, there are some antigens which polyclonally activate a large fraction of the T cells (up to 25%). Examples of superantigens include: Staphylococcal enterotoxins (food poisoning), Staphylococcal toxic shock toxin (toxic shock syndrome), Staphylococcal exfoliating toxins (scalded skin syndrome) and Streptococcal pyrogenic exotoxins (shock). Although the bacterial superantigens are the best studied there are superantigens associated with viruses and other microorganisms as well. The diseases associated with exposure to superantigens are, in part, due to hyper activation of the immune system and subsequent release of biologically active cytokines by activated T cells.

Determinants Recognized by the Innate Immune System

Determinants recognized by components of the innate (nonspecific) immune system differ from those recognized by the adaptive (specific) immune system. Antibodies, and the B and T cell receptors recognize discrete determinants and demonstrate a high degree of specificity, enabling the adaptive immune system to recognize and react to a particular pathogen. In contrast, components of the innate immune system recognize broad molecular patterns found in pathogens but not in the host. Thus, they lack a high degree of specificity seen in the adaptive immune system. The broad molecular patterns recognized by the innate immune system have been called PAMPS (pathogen associated molecular patterns) and the receptors for PAMPS are called PRRs (pattern recognition receptors). A particular PRR can recognize a molecular pattern that may be present on a number of different pathogens enabling the receptor to recognize a variety of different pathogens.

Immunoglobulins - Structure and Function

Immunoglobulin (Ig)

Immunoglobulins are glycoprotein molecules that are produced by plasma cells in response to an immunogen and which function as antibodies. The immunoglobulins derive their name from the finding that they migrate with globular proteins when antibody-containing serum is placed in an electrical field.

General Functions of Immunoglobulins

Antigen Binding: Immunoglobulins bind specifically to one or a few closely related antigens. Each immunoglobulin actually binds to a specific antigenic determinant. Antigen binding by antibodies is the primary function of antibodies and can result in protection of the host. The valency of antibody refers to the number of antigenic determinants that an individual antibody molecule can bind. The valency of all antibodies is at least two and in some instances more.

Effector Functions: Frequently the binding of an antibody to an antigen has no direct biological effect. Rather, the significant biological effects are a consequence of secondary "effector functions" of antibodies. The immunoglobulins mediate a variety of these effector functions.

Usually the ability to carry out a particular effector function requires that the antibody bind to its antigen. Not every immunoglobulin will mediate all effector functions. Such effector functions include:

1. Fixation of complement - This results in lysis of cells and release of biologically active molecules
2. Binding to various cell types - Phagocytic cells, lymphocytes, platelets, mast cells, and basophils have receptors that bind immunoglobulins. This binding can activate the cells to perform some function. Some immunoglobulins also bind to receptors on placental trophoblasts, which results in transfer of the immunoglobulin across the placenta. As a result, the transferred maternal antibodies provide immunity to the fetus and newborn.

Basic Structure of Immunoglobulins

Although different immunoglobulins can differ structurally, they all are built from the same basic units.

Heavy and Light Chains : All immunoglobulins have a four chain structure as their basic unit. They are composed of two identical light chains (23kD) and two identical heavy chains (50-70kD).

Disulfide Bonds:

1. Inter-chain disulfide bonds - The heavy and light chains and the two heavy chains are held together by inter-chain disulfide bonds and by non-covalent interactions The number of inter-chain disulfide bonds varies among different immunoglobulin molecules.
2. Intra-chain disulfide binds - Within each of the polypeptide chains there are also intra-chain disulfide bonds.

Variable (V) and Constant (C) Regions: When the amino acid sequences of many different heavy chains and light chains were compared, it became clear that both the heavy and light chain could be divided into two regions based on variability in the amino acid sequences. These are the:

1. Light Chain - V_L (110 amino acids) and C_L (110 amino acids)
2. Heavy Chain - V_H (110 amino acids) and C_H (330-440 amino acids).

Hinge Region: This is the region at which the arms of the antibody molecule forms a Y. It is called the hinge region because there is some flexibility in the molecule at this point.

Domains: Three dimensional images of the immunoglobulin molecule show that it is not straight. Rather, it is folded into globular regions each of which contains an intra-chain disulfide bond. These regions are called domains.

1. Light Chain Domains - V_L and C_L
2. Heavy Chain Domains - V_{H}, C_{H1} - C_{H3} (or C_{H4}).

Oligosaccharides: Carbohydrates are attached to the C_{H2} domain in most immunoglobulins. However, in some cases carbohydrates may also be attached at other locations.

Structure of the Variable Region

Hypervariable (HVR) or Complementarity Determining Regions (CDR) : Comparisons of the amino acid sequences of the variable regions of immunoglobulins show that most of the variability resides in three regions called the hypervariable regions or the complementarity determining regions. Antibodies with different specificities (i.e. different combining sites) have different complementarity determining regions while antibodies of the exact same specificity have identical complementarity determining regions (*i.e.* CDR is the antibody combining site). Complementarity determining regions are found in both the H and the L chains.

Framework Regions: The regions between the complementarity determining regions in the variable region are called the framework regions. Based on similarities and differences in the framework regions the immunoglobulin heavy and light chain variable regions can be divided into groups and subgroups. These represent the products of different variable region genes.

Immunoglobulin Fragments: Structure/Function Relationships

Immunoglobulin fragments produced by proteolytic digestion have proven very useful in elucidating structure/function relationships in immunoglobulins.

Fab

Digestion with papain breaks the immunoglobulin molecule in the hinge region before the H-H inter-chain disulfide bond. This results in the formation of two identical fragments that contain the light chain and the V_H and C_{H1} domains of the heavy chain.

Antigen binding - These fragments were called the Fab fragments because they contained the antigen binding sites of the antibody. Each Fab fragment is monovalent whereas the original molecule was divalent.

The combining site of the antibody is created by both V_H and V_L. An antibody is able to bind a particular antigenic determinant because it has a particular combination of V_H and V_L. Different combinations of a V_H and V_L result in antibodies that can bind a different antigenic determinants.

Fc

Digestion with papain also produces a fragment that contains the remainder of the two heavy chains each containing a C_{H2} and C_{H3} domain. This fragment was called Fc because it was easily crystallized.

Effector functions - The effector functions of immunoglobulins are mediated by this part of the molecule. Different functions are mediated by the different domains in this fragment. Normally the ability of an antibody to carry out an effector function requires the prior binding of an antigen; however, there are exceptions to this rule.

C. F(ab')$_2$

Treatment of immunoglobulins with pepsin results in cleavage of the heavy chain after the H-H inter-chain disulfide bonds resulting in a fragment that contains both antigen binding sites. This fragment was called F(ab')2 because it is divalent. The Fc region of the molecule is digested into small peptides by pepsin. The F(ab')$_2$ binds antigen but it does not mediate the effector functions of antibodies.

Human Immunoglobulin Classes, Subclasses, Types and Subtypes

Immunoglobulin Classes

The immunoglobulins can be divided into five different classes, based on differences in the amino acid sequences in the constant region of the heavy chains. All immunoglobulins within a given class will have very similar heavy chain constant regions. These differences can be detected by sequence studies or more commonly by serological means (*i.e.* by the use of antibodies directed to these differences).

1. IgG - Gamma heavy chains
2. IgM - Mu heavy chains
3. IgA - Alpha heavy chains
4. IgD - Delta heavy chains
5. IgE - Epsilon heavy chains.

Immunoglobulin Subclasses

The classes of immunoglobulins can de divided into subclasses based on small differences in the amino acid sequences in the constant region of the heavy chains. All immunoglobulins within a subclass will have very similar heavy chain constant region amino acid sequences. Again these differences are most commonly detected by serological means.

1. IgG Subclasses
   a) IgG1 - Gamma 1 heavy chains
   b) IgG2 - Gamma 2 heavy chains
   c) IgG3 - Gamma 3 heavy chains
   d) IgG4 - Gamma 4 heavy chains
2. IgA Subclasses:
   a) IgA1 - Alpha 1 heavy chains
   b) IgA2 - Alpha 2 heavy chains.

Immunoglobulin Types

Immunoglobulins can also be classified by the type of light chain that they have. Light chain types are based on differences in the amino acid sequence in the constant region of the light chain. These differences are detected by serological means.

1. Kappa light chains
2. Lambda light chains.

Immunoglobulin Subtypes

The light chains can also be divided into subtypes based on differences in the amino acid sequences in the constant region of the light chain.

1. Lambda subtypes:
   a) Lambda 1
   b) Lambda 2

c) Lambda 3
d) Lambda 4.

Nomenclature

Immunoglobulins are named based on the class, or subclass of the heavy chain and type or subtype of light chain. Unless it is stated precisely, you should assume that all subclass, types and subtypes are present. IgG means that all subclasses and types are present.

Heterogeneity

Immunoglobulins considered as a population of molecules are normally very heterogeneous because they are composed of different classes and subclasses each of which has different types and subtypes of light chains. In addition, different immunoglobulin molecules can have different antigen binding properties because of different V_H and V_L regions.

Structure and some Properties if IgG Classes and Subclasses

IgG

Structure : All IgG's are monomers (7S immunoglobulin). The subclasses differ in the number of disulfide bonds and length of the hinge region.

Properties : IgG is the most versatile immunoglobulin because it is capable of carrying out all of the functions of immunoglobulin molcecules.

a) IgG is the major Ig in serum - 75% of serum Ig is IgG
b) IgG is the major Ig in extra vascular spaces
c) Placental transfer IgG is the only class of Ig that crosses the placenta. Transfer is mediated by a receptor on placental cells for the Fc region of IgG. Not all subclasses cross equally well; IgG2 does not cross well.
d) Fixes complement - Not all subclasses fix equally well; IgG4 does not fix complement
e) Binding to cells - Macrophages, monocytes, PMNs and some lymphocytes have Fc receptors for the Fc region of IgG. Not all subclasses bind equally well; IgG2 and IgG4 do not bind to Fc receptors. A consequence of binding to the Fc receptors on PMNs, monocytes and macrophages is that the cell can now

internalize the antigen better. The antibody has prepared the antigen for eating by the phagocytic cells. The term opsonin is used to describe substances that enhance phagocytosis. IgG is a good opsonin. Binding of IgG to Fc receptors on other types of cells results in the activation of other functions.

IgM

Structure : IgM normally exists as a pentamer (19S immunoglobulin) but it can also exist as a monomer. In the pentameric form all heavy chains are identical and all light chains are identical. Thus, the valence is theoretically 10. IgM has an extra domain on the mu chain (C_{H4}) and it has another protein covalently bound via a S-S bond called the J chain. This chain functions in polymerization of the molecule into a pentamer.

Properties :

a) IgM is the third most common serum Ig.

b) IgM is the first Ig to be made by the fetus and the first Ig to be made by a virgin B cells when it is stimulated by antigen.

c) As a consequence of its pentameric structure, IgM is a good complement fixing Ig. Thus, IgM antibodies are very efficient in leading to the lysis of microorganisms.

d) As a consequence of its structure, IgM is also a good agglutinating Ig . Thus, IgM antibodies are very good in clumping microorganisms for eventual elimination from the body.

e) IgM binds to some cells via Fc receptors.

f) B cell surface Ig.

Surface IgM exists as a monomer and lacks J chain but it has an extra 20 amino acids at the C-terminus to anchor it into the membrane. Cell surface IgM functions as a receptor for antigen on B cells. Surface IgM is noncovalently associated with two additional proteins in the membrane of the B cell called Ig-alpha and Ig-beta. These additional proteins act as signal transducing molecules since the cytoplasmic tail of the Ig molecule itself is too short to transduce a signal. Contact between surface immunoglobulin and an antigen is required before a signal can be transduced by the Ig-alpha and Ig-beta chains. In the case of T-independent antigens, contact between the antigen and surface immunoglobulin is sufficient to activate B cells to differentiate into antibody secreting plasma cells. However, for T-dependent antigens, a second signal provided by helper T cells is required before B cells are activated.

IgA

Structure : When IgA exits as a dimer, a J chain is associated with it.

When IgA is found in secretions is also has another protein associated with it called the secretory piece or T piece; sIgA is sometimes referred to as 11S immunoglobulin. Unlike the remainder of the IgA which is made in the plasma cell, the secretory piece is made in epithelial cells and is added to the IgA as it passes into the secretions. The secretory piece helps IgA to be transported across mucosa and also protects it from degradation in the secretions.

Properties :

a) IgA is the 2nd most common serum Ig.

b) IgA is the major class of Ig in secretions - tears, saliva, colostrum, mucus. Since it is found in secretions secretory IgA is important in local (mucosal) immunity.

c) Normally IgA does not fix complement, unless aggregated.

d) IgA can binding to some cells - PMN's and some lymphocytes.

IgD

Structure : The structure of IgD is presented. IgD exists only as a monomer.

Properties :

a) IgD is found in low levels in serum; its role in serum uncertain.

b) IgD is primarily found on B cell surfaces where it functions as a receptor for antigen. IgD on the surface of B cells has extra amino acids at C-terminal end for anchoring to the membrane. It also associates with the Ig-alpha and Ig-beta chains.

c) IgD does not bind complement.

IgE

Structure : IgE exists as a monomer and has an extra domain in the constant region.

Properties :

a) IgE is the least common serum Ig since it binds very tightly to Fc receptors on basophils and mast cells even before interacting with antigen.

b) Involved in allergic reactions - As a consequence of its binding to basophils an mast cells, IgE is involved in allergic reactions. Binding of the allergen to the IgE on the cells results in the release of various pharmacological mediators that result in allergic symptoms.

c) IgE also plays a role in parasitic helminth diseases. Since serum IgE levels rise in parasitic diseases, measuring IgE levels is helpful in diagnosing parasitic infections. Eosinophils have Fc receptors for IgE and binding of eosinophils to IgE-coated helminths results in killing of the parasite.

d) IgE does not fix complement.

Clinical Implications of Human Immunoglobulin Classes

IgG

1. Increases in:
   a) Chronic granulomatous infections
   b) Infections of all types
   c) Hyperimmunization
   d) Liver disease
   e) Malnutrition (severe)
   f) Dysproteinemia
   g) Disease associated with hypersensitivity granulomas, dermatologic disorders, and IgG myeloma
   h) Rheumatoid arthritis.
2. Decreases in:
   a) Agammaglobulinemia
   b) Lymphoid aplasia
   c) Selective IgG, IgA deficiency
   d) IgA myeloma
   e) Bence Jones proteinemia
   f) Chronic lymphoblastic leukemia.

IgM

1. Increases (in adults) in:
   a) Waldenström's macroglobulinemia
   b) Trypanosomiasis

c) Actinomycosis
d) Carrión's disease (bartonellosis)
e) Malaria
f) Infectious mononucleosis
g) Lupus erythematosus
h) Rheumatoid arthritis
i) Dysgammaglobulinemia (certain cases).

Note: In the newborn, a level of IgM above 20 ng./dl is an indication of *in utero* stimulation of the immune system and stimulation by the rubella virus, the cytomegalovirus, syphilis, or toxoplasmosis.

2. Decreases in:
   a) Agammaglobulinemia
   b) Lymphoproliferative disorders (certain cases)
   c) Lymphoid aplasia
   d) IgG and IgA myeloma
   e) Dysgammaglobulinemia
   f) Chronic lymphoblastic leukemia.

IgA

1. Increases in:
   a) Wiskott-Aldrich syndrome
   b) Cirrhosis of the liver (most cases)
   c) Certain stages of collagen and other auto-immune disorders such as rheumatoid arthritis and lupus erythematosus
   d) Chronic infections not based on immunologic deficiencies
   e) IgA myeloma.
2. Decreases in:
   a) Hereditary ataxia telangiectasia
   b) Immunologic deficiency states (*e.g.*, dysgammaglobulinemia, congenital and acquired agammaglobulinemia, and hypogammaglobulinemia)
   c) Malabsorption syndromes
   d) Lymphoid aplasia
   e) IgG myeloma
   f) Acute lymphoblastic leukemia
   g) Chronic lymphoblastic leukemia.

IgD

1. Increases in:
   a) Chronic infections
   b) IgD myelomas.

IgE

1. Increases in:
   a) Atopic skin diseases such as eczema
   b) Hay fever
   c) Asthma
   d) Anaphylactic shock
   e) IgE-myeloma.
2. Decreases in:
   a) Congenital agammaglobulinemia
   b) Hypogammaglobulinemia due to faulty metabolism or synthesis of immunoglobulins.

The Structure and Function of Immunoglobulins - Antibodies

Isotypes, Allotypes and Idiotypes

Definition : Isotypes are antigenic determinants that characterize classes and subclasses of heavy chains and types and subtypes of light chains.

If human IgM is injected into a rabbit the rabbit will recognize antigenic determinants on the heavy chain and light chain and make antibodies to them. If that antiserum is absorbed with human IgG the antibodies to the light chain determinants and any determinants in common between human IgM and IgG will be removed and the resulting antiserum will be react only with human IgM.

Indeed, the antibodies will only react with the constant region of the heavy chain. Antibodies to the variable region are rare perhaps because only a few copies of each different variable region are represented in the IgM and thus effective immunization does not occur. The determinants that are recognized by such antibodies are called *isotypic determinants* and the antibodies to those determinants are called *anti-isotypic antibodies*. Each class, subclass, type and subtype of immunoglobulin has its unique set of isotypic determinants.

Location : Heavy chain isotypes are found on the Fc portion of the constant region of the molecule while light chain isotypes are found in the constant region.

Occurrence : Isotypes are found in ALL NORMAL individuals in the species. The prefix Iso means same in all members of the species. Some individuals with immunodeficiencies may lack one or more isotypes but normal individuals have all isotypes.

Importance : Antibodies to isotypes are used for the quantitation of immunoglobulin classes and subclasses in various diseases, in the characterization of B cell leukemia and in the diagnosis of various immunodeficiency diseases.

Allotypes

Definition : Allotypes are antigenic determinants specified by allelic forms of the immunoglobulin genes.

Allotypes represent slight differences in the amino acid sequences of heavy or light chains of different individuals. Even a single amino acid difference can give rise to an allotypic determinant, although in many cases there are several amino acid substitutions that have occurred.

Allotypic differences are detected by using antibodies directed against allotypic determinants. These antibodies can be prepared by injecting the immunoglobulin from one person into another. In practice, however, we obtain anti-allotype antisera from women who have had multiple pregnancies or from people who have received blood transfusions or from some patients with rheumatoid arthritis.

Location : In humans, the allotypic differences are localized to the constant region of the heavy and light chains.

Occurrence : Individual allotypes are found in individual members of a species. All allotypes are not found in all members of the species. The prefix Allo means different in individuals of a species

Antigenic Determinants Created by the Hypervariable Region of an Antibody are Idiotypes

Location

Idiotypes are localized on the Fab fragment of the Ig molecules. Specifically, they are localized at or near the hypervariable regions of the heavy and light chains. In many instances, the actual antigenic determinant (i.e. idiotype) may include some of the framework residues near the hypervariable region. Idiotypes are usually determinants created by both heavy and light chain HVR's although sometimes isolated heavy and light chains will express the idiotype.

Importance

- V region marker - Idiotypes are a useful marker for a particular variable region.
- Regulation of immune responses - There is evidence that immune responses may be regulated by anti-Id antibodies directed against our own Id's.
- Vaccines - In some cases, anti-idiotypic antibodies actually stimulate B cells to make antibody and thus they can be used as a vaccine. This approach is being tried to immunize against highly dangerous pathogens that cannot be safely used as a vaccine.
- Treatment of B cell tumors - Anti-idiotypic antibodies directed against an idiotype on malignant B cells can be used to kill the cells. Killing occurs because of complement fixation or because toxic molecules are attached to the antibodies.

Order of Gene Expression in Immunoglobulin Gene Families

An individual B cell only produces one type of light chain and one class of heavy chain. Since any B cell has both maternal and paternal chromosomes which code for the immunoglobulin genes there must be some orderly way in which a cell expresses its immunoglobulin genes so as to ensure that only one type of light chain and one class of heavy chain is produced.

Heavy Chain

A cell first attempts to rearrange one of its heavy chain genes; in some cells the maternal chromosome is selected and in others the paternal chromosome is selected. If the rearrangement is successful so that a heavy chain is made, then no further rearrangements occur in the heavy chain genes.

If, on the other hand, the first attempt to rearrange the heavy chain genes is unsuccessful (*i.e.* no heavy chain is made), then the cell attempts to rearrange the heavy chain genes on its other chromosome. If the cell is unsuccessful in rearranging the heavy chain genes the second time, it is destined to be eliminated.

Kappa Light Chain

When a cell successfully rearranges a heavy chain gene, it then begins to rearrange one of its *kappa* light chain genes. It is a random event whether the maternal or paternal *kappa* light chain genes are selected. If the rearrangement is unsuccessful (*i.e.* it does not produce a functional *kappa* light chain), then it attempts to rearrange the *kappa* genes on the other chromosome. If a cell successfully rearranges a *kappa* light chain gene, it will be a B cell that makes an immunoglobulin with a *kappa* light chain.

Lambda Light Chain

If a cell is unsuccessful in rearranging both of its *kappa* light chain genes, it then attempts to make a *lambda* light chain. It is a random event whether the maternal or paternal *lambda* light chain genes are selected. If the rearrangement is unsuccessful (*i.e.* it does not produce a functional *lambda* light chain), then it attempts to rearrange the *lambda* genes on the other chromosome. If a cell successfully rearranges a *lambda* light chain gene, it will be a B cell that makes an immunoglobulin with a *lambda* light chain. The orderly sequence of rearrangements in the immunoglobulin gene families explains:

- Why an individual B cell can only produce one kind of immunoglobulin with one kind of heavy and one kind of light chain.
- Why a individual B cell can only make antibodies of one specificity.
- Why there is allelic exclusion in immunoglobulin allotypes at the level of an individual immunoglobulin molecule but co-dominant expression of allotypes in the organism as a whole.

Origin of Antibody Diversity

Antibody diversity refers to the sum total of all the possible antibody specificities that an organism can make. It is estimated that we can make 10^7 - 10^8 different antibody molecules. One of the major questions in immunology has been how can we make so many different antibody molecules. Theories which have attempted to explain the origin of antibody diversity fall into two major categories.

Germ Line Theory

This theory states that we have a different V region gene for each possible antibody we can make.

Somatic Mutation Theory

This theory states that we have only one or a few V region genes and the diversity is generated by somatic mutations which occur in these genes.

Current Concepts

Our current thinking is that both the germ line and somatic mutation theories have some merit. It is thought that antibody diversity is generated by the following mechanisms.

A Large Number of V Genes

There are:

a) 30 *lambda* V genes

b) 300 *kappa* V genes

c) 1000 heavy chain V genes.

V-J and V-D-J Joining

The region where the light chain V gene and J region or the heavy chain V gene and D and J regions come together is in the third hypervariable region. Since it is random which V and which J or D regions come together, there is a lot of diversity that can be generated by V-J and V-D-J joining.

Junctional Diversity (Inaccuracies in V-J and V-D and D-J Recombination)

Recombination between V-J and V-D-J is not always perfect and additional diversity can arise by errors that occur in the recombination event that brings the V region next to the J or D regions or the D region next to the J region. It is estimated that these inaccuracies can triple the diversity generated by V-J and V-D-J joining.

The diversity generated by this mechanism is occurring in the third hypervariable region and thus, is directly affecting the combining site of the antibody.

N Region Insertion

At the junction between D and J segments there is often an insertion of a series of nucleotides which is catalyzed by the enzyme terminal transferase. Terminal transferase catalyzes the random polymerization of nucleotides into DNA without the need for a template. This leads to further diversity in the third hypervariable region.

Somatic Mutation

There is evidence that somatic mutations are occurring in the V gene, particularly in the place that codes for the second hypervariable region. Thus, somatic mutation probably contributes to antibody diversity to some extent.

Combinatorial Association

Any individual B cell has the potential to make any one of the possible heavy chains and any one of the possible light chains. Thus, different combinations of heavy and light chains within an individual B cell adds further diversity.

Multispecificity

Due to cross reactions between antigenic determinants of similar structure an antibody can often react with more than one antigenic determinant. This is termed multispecificity. Multispecificity also contributes to antibody diversity.

Chapter

2

Cytokines and Immunoregulation

Overview

Cytokines are a diverse group of non-antibody proteins that act as mediators between cells. They were initially identified as products of immune cells that act as mediators and regulators of immune processes but many cytokines are now known to be produced by cells other than immune cells and they can have effects on non-immune cells as well. Cytokines are currently being used clinically as biological response modifiers for the treatment of various disorders. The term cytokine is a general term used to describe a large group of proteins but there are other terms that are commonly used to describe particular kinds of cytokines. These include:

- Monokines, cytokines produced by mononuclear phagocytic cells
- Lymphokines, cytokines produced by activated lymphocytes, especially Th cells
- Interleukins, cytokines that act as mediators between leukocytes
- Chemokines, small cytokines primarily responsible for leucocyte migration.

Cytokines function as part of a larger inter-related system of proteins and signaling cascades, the cytokine network. These are complex interactions in which different cells can respond differently to the same cytokine depending upon other signals received by the cell. Cytokine signaling is very flexible and can induce both protective and damaging responses.

One cytokine often influences the synthesis of other cytokines. They can produce cascades, or enhance or suppress production of other cytokines. In addition, they can often influence the action of other cytokines. The effects can be: antagonistic, additive, or synergistic.

Cytokines are not typically stored as preformed proteins. Rather their synthesis is initiated by gene transcription and their mRNAs are short lived. They are produced as needed in immune responses. Genes encoding cytokines can produce variants through alternative splicing to yield proteins with slightly different but biologically significant bioactivities.

Many individual cytokines are produced by many cell types involved in both the innate and adaptive immune response. Individual cytokines also act on many cell types (*i.e.,* they are pleotropic) and in many cases cytokines have similar actions (*i.e.,* they are redundant). Redundancy is due to the nature of the cytokine receptors. Receptors for cytokines are heterodimers (sometimes heterotrimers) that can be grouped into families based on common structural features; one subunit is common to all members of a given family.

- Type 1 cytokine receptors (IL-2R family) are the largest family of cytokine receptors. This family is divided into three subsets based on common components: IL2Rγ, common β, and gp130. These receptors lack intrinsic protein tyrosine kinase activity. Ligand (cytokine) binding leads to receptor dimerization and initiation of intracellular signaling
- Type 2 cytokine receptors (IFNR family) have conserved cysteines in the extracellular domains of the subunits. The extracellular domains also have tandem immunoglobulin-like domains characteristic of this cytokine receptor family. These receptor subunits also have intrinsic tyrosine kinase activity.

Chemokine receptors all have seven transmembrane segments linked to GTP-binding proteins. They are selectively expressed on particular lymphocyte populations and are named based on the family of chemokines to which they bind; CCR (the CC receptor) binds CC chemokines as its ligand while the CXCR binds CXC chemokines as its ligand (chemokines naming convention will be discussed below).

Since the subunit common to all members of the family functions in binding cytokine and in signal transduction, a receptor for one cytokine can often respond to another cytokine in the same family. Thus, an individual lacking IL-2, for example, is not adversely affected because other cytokines (IL-15, IL-9, IL-9, etc.) assume its function. Similarly, a mutation in a cytokine receptor subunit other than the one in common often has little effect.

On the other hand, a mutation in the common subunit has profound effects. For example, a mutation in the gene for the IL-2R gamma subunit causes human X-linked severe combined immunodeficiency (XSCID) characterized by a complete or nearly complete T and B cell defects. Cytokines bind to specific receptors on target cells with high affinity and the cells that respond to a cytokine are either:

- The same cell that secreted cytokine (autocrine)
- A nearby cell (paracrine)
- A distant cell reached through the circulation (endocrine). Cellular responses to cytokines are generally slow (hours) because they require new mRNA and protein synthesis.

Categories of Cytokines

Cytokines can be grouped into different categories based on their functions or their source but it is important to remember that because they can be produced by many different cells and act on many different cells, any attempt to categorize them will be subject to limitations.

Mediators of Natural Immunity (Innate Immune Response)

Cytokines that play a major role in the innate immune system include: TNF-α, IL-1, IL-10, IL-12, type I interferons (IFN-α and IFN-β), IFN-γ, and chemokines.

TNF-α

Tumor necrosis factor alpha is produced by activated macrophages is response to microbes, especially the lipopolysaccharide (LPS) of Gram negative bacteria. It is an important mediator of acute inflammation.

It mediates the recruitment of neutrophils and macrophages to sites of infection by stimulating endothelial cells to produce adhesion molecules and by producing chemokines which are chemotactic cytokines. TNF- α also acts on the hypothalamus to produce fever and it promotes the production of acute phase proteins.

IL-1

Interleukin 1 is another inflammatory cytokine produced by activated macrophages. Its effects are similar to that of TNF-α and it also helps to activate T cells.

IL-10,

Interleukin 10 is produced by activated macrophages and Th2 cells. It is predominantly an inhibitory cytokine. It inhibits production of IFN-γ by Th1 cells, which shifts immune responses toward a Th2 type. It also inhibits cytokine production by activated macrophages and the expression of class II MHC and co-stimulatory molecules on macrophages, resulting in a dampening of immune responses.

IL-12

Interleukin 12 is produced by activated macrophages and dendritic cells. It stimulates the production of IFN-γ and induces the differentiation of Th cells to become Th1 cells. In addition, it enhances the cytolytic functions of Tc and NK cells.

Type I Interferons

Type I interferons (IFN-α and IFN-β) are produced by many cell types and they function to inhibit viral replication in cells. They also increase expression of class I MHC molecules on cells making them more susceptible to killing by CTLs. Type I interferons also activate NK cells.

INF-γ

Interferon gamma is an important cytokine produced by primarily by Th1 cells, although it can also be produced by Tc and NK cells to a lesser extent. It has numerous functions in both the innate and adaptive immune systems.

Chemokines

Chemokines are chemotactic cytokines produced by many kinds of leukocytes and other cell types. They represent a large family of molecules that function to recruit leukocytes to sites of infection and play a role in lymphocyte trafficking by determining which cells will cross the epithelium and where they are directed to go.

There are four families of chemokines based on spacing of conserved cysteine. Two examples are the β-chemokines which have a CXC structure (two cysteines with a different amino acid in between) and the â-chemokines which have a CC structure (two neighboring cysteines). Individual chemokines (within the same family) often bind more than one receptor.

Mediators of Adaptive Immunity

Cytokines that play a major role in the adaptive immune system include: IL-2, IL-4, IL-5, TGF-α, IL-10 and IFN-β.

IL-2

Interleukin 2 is produced by Th cells, although it can also be produced by Tc cells to a lesser extent. It is the major growth factor for T cells. It also promotes the growth of B cells and can activate NK cells and monocytes. IL-2 acts on T cells in an autocrine fashion. Activation of T cells results in expression of IL-2R and the production of IL-2. The IL-2 binds to the IL-R and promotes cell division. When the T cells are no longer being stimulated by antigen.

IL-4

Interleukin 4 is produced by macrophages and Th2 cells. It stimulates the development of Th2 cells from naïve Th cells and it promotes the growth of differentiated Th2 cells resulting in the production of an antibody response. It also stimulates Ig class switching to the IgE isotype.

IL-5

Interleukin 5 is produced by Th2 cells and it functions to promote the growth and differentiation of B cells and eosinophiles. It also activates mature eosinophiles.

TGF-β

Transforming growth factor beta is produced by T cells and many other cell types. It is primarily an inhibitory cytokine. It inhibits the proliferation of T cells and the activation of macrophages. It also acts on PMNs and endothelial cells to block the effects of pro-inflammatory cytokines.

Stimulators of Hematopoesis

Some cytokines stimulate the differentiation of hematopoetic cells. These include GM-CSF which promotes the differentiation of bone marrow progenitors, M-CSF, which promotes growth and differentiation of progenitors into monocytes and macrophages and G-CSF, which promotes production of PMNs.

Interleukin 17

IL-17, is proinflammatory cytokine approximately 150 amino acids long. The IL-17, family includes six members which share sequence homology but differential tissue expression. IL-17 is produced by Th17 cells and its over expression has been associated with autoimmune disease including multiple sclerosis, rheumatoid arthritis, and inflammatory bowel disease.

Cytokine Networks

Although the focus of most research has been on the production and action of cytokines on cells of the immune system, it is important to remember that many of them have effects on other cells and organ systems. In fact, the cytokine network is rather complex and represents a series of overlapping and inter-related connections amongst cytokines. Within this network, one cytokine may induce or suppress its own synthesis, induce or suppress the synthesis of other cytokines, induce or suppress synthesis of cytokine receptors (both its own and other cytokine receptors), and antagonize or synergize with other cytokines.

Immunoregulation

The magnitude of an immune response is determined by the balance between antigen-driven activation of lymphocytes and negative regulatory influences that prevent or dampen the response. Regulatory mechanisms can act at the recognition, activation or effector phases of an immune response. Examples of regulation that have already been discussed include:

- Recognition of antigen in the absence of co-stimulation resulting in anergy
- Recognition of antigen with CTLA-4 engagement of B7 resulting in down regulation of T cell activation
- Cytokines with stimulatory or inhibitory activities on immune cells
- Idiotype/anti-idiotype interactions leading to stimulation or inhibition of immune responses
- Dose and route of antigen exposure can induce differential Th responses which in one case can protect and in another can tolerize.

Regulation by Antibody

Soluble antibody can compete with antigen receptors on B cells and block or prevent B cell activation. In addition antigen antibody complexes can bind to Fc receptors on B cells, sending an inhibitory signal to B cells.

In this case the regulation is occurring at the recognition level. In addition, antigen-antibody complexes can bind to Fc receptors on B cells, sending an inhibitory signal to B cells. Here regulation occurs at the activation level.

Antibody can also regulate activation (enhance) by maintaining a source of antigen for APC. In this case, antibody binds antigen forming an immune complex which binds and activated the complement system. Complement activation allows for ligation to the complement receptor on the APC.

Regulation by Cytokines

Cytokines are positive or negative regulators. They act at many stages of the immune response, but their activity is dependent upon the other cytokines present in the micro environment as well as receptor expression on effector cells. Cytokines regulate the type and extent of the immune response generated.

Regulation by Regulatory T Cells (Tregs)

Regulatory T cells (Tregs) are a recently described populations of cells that can regulate immune responses. They do not prevent initial T cell activation; rather, they inhibit a sustained response and prevent chronic and potentially damaging responses. They do not have characteristics of Th1, Th2 or TH17 cells but they can suppress both Th1 and Th2 responses.

Naturally Occurring Tregs

The thymus gives rise to CD4+/CD25+/Foxp3+ cells that functions as Tregs. These Tregs suppress immune responses in a cell contact dependent manner but the mechanism of suppression has not been established.

Induced Tregs

In the periphery some T cells are induced to become Tregs by antigen and either IL-10, or TGF-β. Tregs induced by IL-10 are CD4+/CD25+/Foxp3- and are referred to as Tr1 cells.

These cells suppress immune responses by secretion of IL10. Tregs induced by TGF-β are CD4+/CD25+/Foxp3+ and are referred to as induced Tregs. These cells suppress by secretion of TGF-β

CD8+ Tregs

Some CD8+ cells can also be induced by antigen and IL-10 to become a Treg cell. These cells are CD8+/Foxp3+ and they suppress by a cell contact dependent mechanism or by secretion of cytokines. These cells have been demonstrated *in vitro* but it is not known whether they exist *in vivo*.

Genetic Factors Influencing Immunoregulation

MHC-linked genes help control response to infection. Certain HLA haplotypes are associated with individuals who are responders or nonresponder, those who are susceptible or resistant.

Non-MHC genes are also involved in immunoregulation. An example is a gene related to macrophage activity encoding a transporter protein involved in transport of nitrite (NO2-) into the phagolysosome, natural resistance-associated macrophage protein-1 (Nramp1). Polymorphisms in this gene could change the activity of macrophages.

Cytokine, chemokine, and their receptors are involved in immunoregulation as discussed above. Polymorphisms in the genes encoding these, in particular the receptors, have been shown to correlate to susceptibility to infection or generation of auto-immune disease.

Immunization

Immunization is a means of providing specific protection against many common and damaging pathogens by stimulating an organism's immune system to either produce humoral antibodies against the pathogen (or toxins produced by the pathogen) or T cells that can provide cell-mediated immunity.

The type of immunity that is needed to neutralize a specific pathogen depends on the site of the pathogen and the mechanism of its pathogenesis. For example, some pathogens produce disease by secreting exotoxins. If this is the case, the only immune mechanism effective against the organism would be neutralizing antibodies that prevent exotoxin binding to the appropriate receptor on its target cell and promoting its clearance and degradation by phagocytes.

If the pathogen produces disease by other means, an antibody will have to react with the pathogen itself and eliminate it either by complement-mediated lysis or phagocytosis and intracellular killing. However, if the pathogenic organism is localized intracellularly, it will not be accessible to antibodies and the cell harboring it will have to be destroyed instead; only then could antibody have any effect on the pathogen. Most viruses, together with intracellular bacteria and protozoa, are examples of such pathogens.

In this case, the harboring cells can be destroyed by elements of cell-mediated immunity or, if they cause the infected cell to express unique antigens recognizable by antibody, antibody-dependent and complement-mediated killing of the infected cell can expose the pathogen to elements of humoral immunity. It is also possible for cells harboring intracellular pathogen to be activated to kill the pathogen. Such is clearly not the case with pathogens that have the capability of surviving within phagocytic cells.

Specific immunity can result from either passive or active immunization and both modes of immunization can occur by natural or artificial processes.

Passive Immunity

Immunity can be acquired, without the immune system being challenged with an antigen. This is done by transfer of serum or gamma-globulins from an immune donor to a non-immune individual. Alternatively, immune cells from an immunized individual may be used to transfer immunity. Passive immunity may be acquired naturally or artificially.

Naturally Acquired Passive Immunity

Immunity is transferred from mother to fetus through placental transfer of IgG or colostral transfer of IgA.

Artificially Acquired Passive Immunity

Immunity is often artificially transferred by injection with gamma-globulins from other individuals or gamma-globulin from an immune animal. Passive transfer of immunity with immune globulins or gamma-globulins is used in numerous acute situations of infection (diphtheria, tetanus, measles, rabies, etc.), poisoning (insects, reptiles, botulism), and as a prophylactic measure (hypogammaglobulinemia). In these situations, gamma-globulins of human origin are preferable, although specific antibodies raised in other species are effective and used in some cases (poisoning, diphtheria, tetanus, gas gangrene, botulism). While this form of immunization has the advantage of providing immediate protection, heterologous gamma-globulins are effective for only a short duration and often result in pathological complications (serum sickness) and anaphylaxis. Homologous immunoglobulins also carry the risk of transmitting hepatitis and HIV.

Passive transfer of cell-mediated immunity can also be accomplished in certain diseases (cancer, immunodeficiency). However, it is difficult to find histocompatible (matched) donors and there is severe risk of graft versus host disease.

Active Immunity

This refers to immunity produced by the body following exposure to antigens.

Naturally Acquired Active Immunity

Exposure to various pathogens leads to sub-clinical or clinical infections which result in a protective immune response against these pathogens.

Artificially Acquired Active Immunity

Immunization may be achieved by administering live or dead pathogens or their components. Vaccines used for active immunization consist of live (attenuated) organisms, killed whole organisms, microbial components or secreted toxins (which have been detoxified).

Live Vaccines

The first live vaccine was cowpox virus introduced by Edward Jenner as a vaccine for smallpox; however, variolation (innoculation using pus from a patient with a mild case of smallpox) has been in use for over a thousand years.

Live vaccines are used against a number of viral infections (polio (Sabin vaccine), measles, mumps, rubella, chicken pox, hepatitis A, yellow fever, *etc.*). The only example of live bacterial vaccine is one against tuberculosis (*Mycobacterium bovis*: Bacille Calmette-Guerin vaccine: BCG). This is used in many African, European and Asian countries but not in the United States. Whereas many studies have shown the efficacy of BCG vaccine, a number of studies also cast doubt on its benefits.

Live vaccines normally produce self-limiting non-clinical infections and lead to subsequent immunity, both humoral and cell-mediated, the latter being essential for intracellular pathogens. However, they carry a serious risk of causing overt disease in immunocompromised individuals. Furthermore, since live vaccines are often attenuated (made less pathogenic) by passage in animals or thermal mutation, they can revert to their pathogenic form and cause serious illness. It is for this reason that live polio (Sabin) vaccine, which was used for many years, has been replaced in many countries by the inactivated (Salk) vaccine.

Killed Vaccines

Killed (heat, chemical or UV irradiation) viral vaccines include those for polio (Salk vaccine), influenza, rabies, influenza, rabies, etc. Most bacterial vaccines are killed organisms (typhoid, cholera, plague, pertussis, *etc.*).

Sub-unit Vaccines

Some anti-bacterial vaccines utilize purified cell wall components (haemophilus, pertussis, meningococcus, pneumococcus, etc.). Some viral vaccines (hepatitis-B, *etc.*) consist of purified antigenic proteins manufactured after expression from a gene cloned into a suitable vector (*e.g.*, yeast). When the pathogenic mechanism of an agent involves a toxin, a modified form of the toxin (toxoid, which has lost its toxicity while remaining immunogenic) is used as a vaccine (*e.g.*, diphtheria, tetanus, cholera). These subunit vaccines are designed to reduce the toxicity problems. Each type of vaccine has its own advantages and disadvantages.

Subunit vaccines may consist of proteins or polysaccharides. Since polysaccharides are relatively weak T-independent antigens, and produce only IgM responses without immunologic memory, they are made more immunogenic and T-dependent by conjugation with proteins (e.g., haemophilus, meningococcus, pneumococcus, etc.).

Other Novel Vaccines

A number of novel approaches to active immunization are in the investigative stage and are used only experimentally. These include anti-idiotype antibodies, DNA vaccines and immunodominant peptides (recognized by the MHC molecules) and may be available in the future.

- Anti-idiotype antibodies against polysaccharide antibodies produce long lasting immune responses with immunologic memory.
- DNA vaccines (viral peptide genes cloned into vectors) must be injected. They transfect host cells and consequently produce a response similar to that produced against live-attenuated viruses (both cell-mediated and humoral). Several anti-HIV DNA vaccines have been developed but none has so far shown much efficacy.

- Immunodominant peptides are simple and easy to prepare and, when incorporated into MHC polymers, can provoke both humoral and cell mediated responses.

Adjuvants

Weaker antigens may be rendered more immunogenic by the addition of other chemicals. Such chemicals are known as adjuvants. There are many biological and chemical substances that have been used in experimental conditions. However, only aluminum salts (alum) are approved for human use and it is incorporated in DTP vaccine.

Furthermore, pertussis itself has adjuvant effects. Adjuvants used experimentally include mixtures of oil and detergents, with (Freund's complete adjuvant) or without (Freund's incomplete adjuvant) certain bacteria. Bacteria most often used in an adjuvant are Mycobacteria (BCG) and Nocardia. In some instances, sub-cellular fractions of these bacteria can also be used effectively as adjuvants.

Newer adjuvant formulations include synthetic polymers and oligonucleotides. Most adjuvants recognize TOLL-like receptors, thus activating mononuclear phagocytes and inducing selective cytokines that can enhance Th1 or Th2 responses, depending on the nature of the adjuvant.

The protective immunity conferred by a vaccine may be life-long (measles, mumps, rubella, small pox, tuberculosis, yellow fever, etc.) or may last as little as a few months (cholera). The primary immunization may be given at the age of 2 to 3 months (diphtheria, pertussis, tetanus, polio), or 13 to 15 months (mumps, measles, rubella). The currently recommended schedule for routine immunization in the United States (recommended by CDC and AIP) is summarized. This schedule is revised on a yearly basis or as need by the CDC Advisory Committee on Immunization Practice (AICP).

Prophylactic Versus Therapeutic Immunization

Most vaccines are given prophylactically, i.e. prior to exposure to the pathogen. However, some vaccines can be administered therapeutically, i.e. post exposure (e.g., rabies virus). The effectiveness of this mode of immunization depends on the rate of replication of the pathogen, incubation period and the pathogenic mechanism. For this reason, only a booster shot with tetanus is sufficient if the exposure to the pathogen is within less than 10 years and if the exposure is minimal (wounds are relatively superficial). In a situation where the pathogen has a short incubation period, only a small amount of pathogenic molecules could be fatal (e.g., tetanus and diphtheria); therefore both passive and active post exposure immunization are essential.

This is also the case when a bolus of infection is relatively large. Passive prophylactic immunization is also normal in cases of defects in the immune system, such as hypogammaglobulinemias.

Adverse Effects of Immunization

Active immunization may cause fever, malaise and discomfort. Some vaccine may also cause joint pains or arthritis (rubella), convulsions, that may sometimes be fatal (pertussis), or neurological disorders (influenza). Allergies to eggs may develop as a consequence of viral vaccines produced in eggs (measles, mumps, influenza, yellow fever). Booster shots result in more pronounced inflammatory effects than the primary immunization.

The serious side effects have been documented after use of the DTP vaccine. Most of these were attributable to the whole pertussis component of the vaccine and have been eliminated by the use of an acellular pertussis preparation.

Table : *Approximate rates of adverse event occurring within 48 hours DTP vaccination*

Event	***Frequency Local***
redness, swelling, pain	1 in 2-3 doses
Mild/moderate systemic	
fever, drowsiness, fretfulness	1 in 2-3 doses
vomiting, anorexia	1 in 5-15 doses
More serious systemic	
persistent crying, fever	1 in 100-300 doses
collapse, convulsions	1 in 1750 doses
acute encephalopathy	1 in 100,000 doses
permanent neurological deficit	1 in 300,000 doses

MHC: Genetics and Role in Transplantation

Definitions

- Histocompatibility (transplantation) antigens

  Antigens on tissues and cells that determine their rejection when grafted between two genetically different individuals

- Major histocompatibility (MHC) antigens

  Histocompatibility antigens that cause a very strong immune response and are most important in rejection
- MHC complex

  Group of genes on a single chromosome encoding the MHC antigens
- HLA (human leukocyte antigens)

  MHC antigens of man (first detected on leukocytes)
- H-2 antigens

  MHC antigens of mouse.

Types of Graft

- Xenograft

  Grafts between members of different species (also known as heterologous, xenogeneic or heterografts)
- Allograft

  Grafts between two members of the same species (also known as allogeneic or homograft)
- Isograft

  Grafts between members of the same species with identical genetic makeup (identical twins or inbred animals)
- Haplotype

  A group of genes on a single chromosome.

Principles of Transplantation

An immunocompetent host recognizes the foreign antigens on grafted tissues (or cells) and mounts an immune response which results in rejection. On the other hand, if an immunocompromised host is grafted with foreign immunocompetent lymphoid cells, the immunoreactive T-cells in the graft recognize the foreign antigens on the host tissue, leading to damage of the host tissue.

Host-versus-graft-reaction

The duration of graft survival follows the order, xeno- < allo- < iso- = auto- graft. The time of rejection also depends on the antigenic disparity between the donors and recipient. MHC antigens are the major contributors in rejection, but the minor histocompatibility antigens also play a role. Rejection due to disparity in several minor histocompatibility antigens may be as quick or quicker than rejection mediated by an MHC antigen. As in other immune responses, there is immunological memory and secondary response in graft rejection. Thus, once a graft is rejected by a recipient, a second graft from the same donor, or a donor with the same histocompatibility antigens, will be rejected in a much shorter time.

Graft-versus-host (GVH) Reaction

Histocompatible lymphoid cells, when injected into an immunocompromised host, are readily accepted. However, the immunocompetent T lymphocytes among the grafted cells recognize the alloantigens and, in response, they proliferate and progressively cause damage to the host tissues and cells. This condition is known as graft-versus-host (GVH) disease and is often fatal.

Common manifestations of GVH reaction are diarrhea, erythema, weight loss, malaise, fever, joint pains, etc. and ultimately death.

The MHC Gene Complex

The MHC complex contains a number of genes that control several antigens, most of which influence allograft rejection. These antigens (and their genes) can be divided into three major classes: class I, class II and class III.

The class I and class II antigens are expressed on cells and tissues whereas as class III antigens are represented on proteins in serum and other body fluids (e.g. C4, C2, factor B, TNF). Antigens of class III gene products have no role in graft rejection.

Human MHC

The human MHC is located on chromosome 6.

Class I MHC

The class I gene complex contains three major loci, B, C and A and other undefined minor loci. Each major locus codes for a polypeptide; the alpha-chain that contains antigenic determinants, is polymorphic (has many alleles). It associates with beta-2 microglobulin (beta-chain), encoded by a gene outside the MHC complex, and expressed on the cell surface.

Without the beta-2 microglobulin, the class I antigen will not be expressed on the cell surface. Individuals with a defective beta-2 microglobulin gene do not express any class I antigen and hence have a deficiency of cytotoxic T cells.

Class II MHC

The class II gene complex also contains at least three loci, DP, DQ and DR; each of these loci codes for one alpha- and one beta-chain polypeptide which associate together to form the class II antigens. Like the class I antigens, the class II antigens are also polymorphic. The DR locus may contain more than one, possibly four, functional beta-chain genes.

Mouse MHC

The mouse MHC is located on chromosome 17.

Class I MHC

This consists of two major loci, K and D. Unlike the human MHC, the mouse class I gene complexes loci are not together but they are separated by class II and class III genes.

Class II MHC

The class II gene complex contains two loci, A and E, each of which code for one alpha and one beta chain polypeptide, which form one class II molecule. The mouse class II gene complex is also known as the I region and the genes in this complex are referred to as Ir (immune response) genes since they determine the magnitude of immune responsiveness of different mouse strains to certain antigens. Products of the A and E loci are also termed IA and IE antigens, collectively known as Ia antigens.

MHC Antigens

Nomenclature

HLA specificities are identified by a letter for locus and a number (A1, B5, *etc.*) and the haplotypes are identified by individual specificities (e.g., A1, B7, Cw4, DP5, DQ10, DR8). Specificities which are defined by genomic analysis (PCR), are names with a letter for the locus and a four digit number (e.g. A0101, B0701, C0401 etc). Specificities of mouse MHC (H-2) are identified by a number. Since laboratory mice are inbred, each strain is homozygous and has a unique haplotype. The MHC haplotype in these strains is designated by a 'small' letter (a, b, d, k, q, s, *etc.*); for example, the MHC haplotype of Balb/c mice is $H2^d$.

Inheritance

MHC genes are inherited as a group (haplotype), one from each parent. Thus, a heterozygous human inherits one paternal and one maternal haplotype, each containing three class-I (B, C and A) and three class II (DP, DQ and DR) loci. A heterozygous individual will inherit a maximum of 6 class I specificities. Similarly, the individual will also inherit DP and DQ genes and express both parental antigens. Since the class II MHC molecule consists of two chains (alpha and beta), with some antigenic determinants (specificities) on each chain, and DR alpha- and beta-chains can associate in ether *cis* (both from the same parent) or *trans* (one from each parent) combinations, an individual can have additional DR specificities.

Also, there are more than one functional DR beta-chain genes. Hence, many DR specificities can be found in any one individual.

Crossover

Haplotypes, normally, are inherited intact and hence antigens encoded by different loci are inherited together (e.g., A2; B27; Cw2; DPw6; DQw9; DRw2). However, on occasions, there is crossing over between two parental chromosomes, thereby resulting in new recombinant haplotypes.

Thus, any one specificity encoded by one locus may combine with specificities from other loci. This results in vast heterogeneity in the MHC make-up in a given population.

MHC Antigen Expression on Cells

MHC antigens are expressed on the cell surface in a co-dominant manner: products of both parental genes are found on the same cells. However, not all cells express both class I and class II antigens. While class I antigens are expressed on all nucleated cells and platelets (and red blood cells in the mouse), the expression of class II antigens is more selective. They are expressed on B lymphocytes, a proportion of macrophages and monocytes, skin associated (Langerhans) cells, dendritic cells and occasionally on other cells.

MHC Detection by Serological Test

The MHC class I antigens are detected by serological assays (Ab and C). Tissue typing sera for the HLA were obtained, in the past, from multiparous women who were exposed to the child's paternal antigens during parturition and subsequently developed antibodies to these antigens.

More recently, they are produced by monoclonal antibody technology. With most laboratories switching to PCR for tissue typing, the use of serology is rapidly diminishing.

MHC Detection by Mixed Leukocyte Reaction (MLR)

It has been observed that lymphocytes from one donor, when cultured with lymphocytes from an unrelated donor, are stimulated to proliferate. It has been established that this proliferation is primarily due to a disparity in the class II MHC (DR) antigens and T cells of one individual interact with allogeneic class-II MHC antigen bearing cells (B cells, dendritic cells, langerhans cells, etc.). This reactivity was termed mixed leukocyte reaction (MLR) and has been used for studying the degree of histocompatibility.

In this test, the test lymphocytes (responder cells) are mixed with irradiated or mitomycin C treated leukocytes from the recipient, containing B-lymphocytes and monocytes (stimulator cells). The cells are cultured for 4 6 days. The responder T cells will recognize the foreign class II antigens found on the donor and undergo transformation (DNA synthesis and enlargement: blastogenesis) and proliferation (mitogenesis). The T cells that respond to foreign class II antigens are typically CD4+ TH-1 type cells. These changes are recorded by the addition of radioactive (tritiated, 3H) thymidine into the culture and monitoring its incorporation into DNA.

Generation of Cytotoxic T Lymphocytes

Another consequence of the MHC antigen and T cell interaction is the induction of cytotoxic T-lymphocytes. When T-lymphocytes are cultured in the presence of allogeneic lymphocytes, in addition to undergoing mitosis (MLR), they also become cytotoxic to cells of the type that stimulated MLR. Thus, T-lymphocytes of 'x' haplotype cultured over 5 - 7 days with B lymphocytes of 'y' haplotype will undergo mitosis and the surviving T-lymphocytes become cytotoxic to cells of the 'y' haplotype. The induction of mitosis in MLR requires disparity of only class II antigens whereas the induction of cytotoxic T-lymphocytes (CTL) requires disparity of both class I and class II antigens. However, once cytotoxic cells have been induced, the effector cytotoxic cells recognize only class I antigens to cause cytotoxicity.

Allograft Rejection

The clinical significance of the MHC is realized in organ transplantation. Cells and tissues are routinely transplanted as a treatment for a number of diseases. However, reaction of the host against allo-antigens of the graft (HVG) results in its rejection and is the major obstacle in organ transplantation. The rejection time of a graft may vary with the antigenic nature of the graft and the immune status of the host and is determined by the immune mechanisms involved.

Hyper-acute Rejection

This occurs in instances when the recipient has preformed high titer antibodies. A graft may show signs of rejection within minutes to hours due to immediate reaction of antibodies and complement.

Accelerated (2nd set; Secondary) Rejection

Transplantation of a second graft, which shares a significant number of antigenic determinants with the first one, results in a rapid (2 - 5 days) rejection. It is due to presence of T-lymphocytes sensitized during the first graft rejection. Accelerated rejection is mediated by immediate production of lymphokines, activation of monocytes and macrophages, and induction of cytotoxic lymphocytes.

Acute (1st Set; Primary) Rejection

The normal reaction that follows the first grafting of a foreign transplant takes 1 - 3 weeks. This is known as acute rejection and is mediated by T lymphocytes sensitized to class I and class II antigens of the allograft, elicitation of lymphokines and activation of monocytes and macrophages.

Chronic Rejection

Some grafts may survive for months or even years, but suddenly exhibit symptoms of rejection. This is referred to as chronic rejection, the mechanism of which is not entirely clear. The hypotheses are that this may be due infection, causes which led to failure of the first organ, loss of tolerance induced by the graft, etc.

Fetus as an Allograft

The fetus in an out-bred mammalian species bears antigens derived from both the father and the mother. Thus, truly, the fetus is an allograft and the mother should normally recognize the fetus as foreign and reject the fetus. Nonetheless, such rejections seldom occur. Thus, mammals have adapted in a way that allows implantation of their embryos in the mother's womb and their subsequent survival. There are multiple mechanisms that play a role, of which the most important being the unique structure and function of placenta.

Immunologically Privileged Sites and Tissues

There are certain locations in the body in which allografts are not readily rejected. These include the brain, anterior chamber of the eye, testis, renal tubule, uterus, etc. This stems from the fact that such sites may lack of good lymphatic drainage. Also, such tissues may express molecules such as Fas ligand that kills any immune cell that may come in contact with these tissues. Additionally, such tissues, may have other immune suppressor mechanisms. Similarly, there are some tissues that can be transplanted without matching and without being rejected. Such tissues are called immunologically privileged tissues. Corneal graft is an excellent example that enjoys the highest success rate of any form of organ transplantation. The low incidence of graft rejection is impressive despite the fact that HLA antigen matching of donor and recipient is not normally performed. There are many explanations as to why such grafts are accepted. The avascularity of the graft bed prevents corneal alloantigens from reaching the regional lymphoid tissues. Also, the corneal antigens may be masked. Together, such mechanisms fail to activate the immune system of the recipient.

Procedures to Enhance Graft Survival

In clinical practice, the most successful transplantation programs have been with kidneys and corneas. However, other organs are being transplanted with increasing frequency. The success in these programs has been due to a better understanding of immunological mechanisms, definition of MHC antigens and development of more effective immunosuppressive agents.

Donor Selection

Based on extensive experiences with renal transplants, certain guidelines can be followed in donor selection and recipient preparation for most organ transplants. The most important in donor selection is the MHC identity with the recipient; an identical twin is the ideal donor. Grafts from an HLA-matched sibling have 95-100% chance of success. One haplotype-identical parent or sibling must match at the HLA D region. A two haplotype-distinct donor with a reasonable match for D-region antigen can also be used. Organs from a two or one DR matched cadaver have been used also with some success. In every case, an ABO compatibility is essential.

Recipient Preparation

The recipient must be infection-free and must not be hypertensive. One to five transfusions of 100-200 ml whole blood from the donor at 1-2 week intervals improves the graft survival and is practiced when possible.

Immunosuppression

Immunosuppressive therapy is most essential part of allo-transplantation. The most recent and effective family of agents is cyclosporin A, FK-506 (tacrolimus) and rapamycin. Cyclosporin A and FK506 inhibit IL-2 synthesis following Ag-receptor binding whereas rapamycin interferes with signal transduction following IL2 - IL2 receptor interaction. Thus, all three agents block T cell proliferation in response to antigen. Whole body irradiation is used in leukemia patients before bone marrow transplantation. Antisera against T cells (anti-thymocyte globulin: ATG) or their surface antigens (CD3, CD4, CD45 on activated T-cells, CD25:IL-2 receptors) are being used also to achieve immunosuppression.

Strategies for Bone Marrow Transplantation

In bone marrow transplantation, the most crucial factor in donor selection is class II MHC compatibility. Once again an identical twin is the ideal donor. From poorly matched grafts, T lymphocytes can be removed using monoclonal antibodies. The recipient must be immunosuppressed. Malignant cells must be eliminated from the recipient blood (in case of blood-borne malignancies). Methotrexate, cyclosporin and prednisone are often used to control GVH disease.

Other Grafts

Corneal grafts do not contain D region antigens and consequently survival is frequent. Small grafts are better and corticosteroids are helpful. Skin allografts have a very poor success rate and immunosuppressive therapy is relatively ineffective. Nevertheless, they are often used to provide a temporary covering to promote healing in severe skin damage. Indeed, there will be no rejection if the host and donor are perfectly matched (identical twins) or the recipient is tolerant to the donor MHC antigens (bone marrow chimeras).

MHC Association with Diseases

A number of diseases have been found to occur at a higher frequency in individuals with certain MHC haplotypes. Most prominent among these are ankylosing spondylitis (B27), celiac disease (DR3) and Reiter's syndrome (B27). Other diseases associated with different specificities of the MHC. No definite reason is known for this association. However, several hypotheses have been proposed: antigenic similarity between pathogens and MHC, antigenic hypo- and hyper-responsiveness controlled by the class II genes are included among them.

Tolerance and Autoimmunity

Tolerance

Tolerance refers to the *specific* immunological non-reactivity to an antigen resulting from a previous exposure to the same antigen. While the most important form of tolerance is non-reactivity to self antigens, it is possible to induce tolerance to non-self antigens. When an antigen induces tolerance, it is termed tolerogen.

Tolerance to Self Antigens

We normally do not mount a strong immune response against our own (self) antigens, a phenomenon called self-tolerance. When the immune system recognizes a self antigen and mounts a strong response against it, auto-immune disease develops.

Nonetheless, the immune system has to recognize self-MHC to mount a response against a foreign antigen. Thus, the immune system is constantly challenged to discriminate self vs non-self and mediate the right response.

Induction of Tolerance to Non-self

Tolerance can also be induced to non-self (foreign) antigens by modifying the antigen, by injecting the antigen through specific routes such as oral, administering the antigen when the immune system is developing, etc. Certain bacteria and viruses have devised clever ways to induce tolerance so that the host does not kill these microbes. Ex: Patients with lepromatous type of leprosy do not mount an immune response against *Mycobacterium leprae*.

Tolerance to Tissues and Cells

Tolerance to tissue and cell antigens can be induced by injection of hemopoietic (stem) cells in neonatal or severely immunocompromised (by lethal irradiation or drug treatment) animals. Also, grafting of allogeneic bone marrow or thymus in early life results in tolerance to the donor type cells and tissues. Such animals are known as chimeras. These findings are of significant practical application in bone marrow grafting.

Tolerance to Soluble Antigens

A state of tolerance to a variety of T-dependent and T-independent antigens has been achieved in various experimental models. Based on these observations it is clear that a number of factors determine whether an antigen will stimulate an immune response or tolerance.

Immunologic Features of Tolerance

Tolerance is different from non-specific immunosuppression and immunodeficiency. It is an active antigen-dependent process in response to the antigen. Like immune response, tolerance is specific and like immunological memory, it can exist in T-cells, B cells or both and like immunological memory, tolerance at the T cell level is longer lasting than tolerance at the B cell level.

Induction of tolerance in T cells is easier and requires relatively smaller amounts of tolerogen than tolerance in B cells. Maintenance of immunological tolerance requires persistence of antigen. Tolerance can be broken naturally (as in auto-immune diseases) or artificially (as shown in experimental animals, by x-irradiation, certain drug treatments and by exposure to cross reactive antigens).

Tolerance may be induced to all epitopes or only some epitopes on an antigen and tolerance to a single antigen may exist at the B cell level or T cell level or at both levels.

Mechanism of Tolerance Induction

The exact mechanism of induction and maintenance of tolerance is not fully understood. Experimental data, however, point to several possibilities.

Clonal Deletion

T and B lymphocytes during development come across self antigens and such cells undergo clonal deletion through a process known as apoptosis or programmed cell death. For example, T cells that develop in the thymus first express neither CD4 nor CD8. Such cells next acquire both CD4 and CD8 called double-positive cells and express low levels of αβ TCR. Such cells undergo positive selection after interacting with class I or class II MHC molecules expressed on cortical epithelium.

During this process, cells with low affinity for MHC are positively selected. Unselected cells die by apoptosis, a process called "death by neglect". Next, the cells loose either CD4 or CD8. Such T cells then encounter self-peptides presented by self MHC molecules expressed on dendritic cells. Those T cells with high affinity receptors for MHC + self-peptide undergo clonal deletion also called negative selection through induction of apoptosis. Any disturbance in this process can lead to escape of auto-reactive T-cells that can trigger auto-immune disease. Likewise, differentiating early B cells when they encounter self-antigen, cell associated or soluble, undergo deletion. Thus, clonal deletion plays a key role in ensuring tolerance to self antigen.

Peripheral Tolerance

The clonal deletion is not a fool proof system and often T and B cells fail to undergo deletion and therefore such cells can potentially cause auto-immune disease once they reach the peripheral lymphoid organs. Thus, the immune system has devised several additional check points so that tolerance can be maintained.

Activation-induced Cell Death

T cells upon activation not only produce cytokines or carryout their effector functions but also die through programmed cell death or apoptosis. In this process, the death receptor (Fas) and its ligand (FasL) play a crucial role.

Thus, normal T cells express Fas but not FasL. Upon activation, T cells express FasL which binds to Fas and triggers apoptosis by activation of caspase-8. The importance of Fas and FasL is clearly demonstrated by the observation that mice with mutations in Fas (lpr mutation) or FasL (gld mutation) develop severe lymphoproliferative and auto-immune disease and die within 6 months while normal mice live up to 2 years. Similar mutations in these apoptotic genes in humans leads to a lymphoproliferative disease called autoimmune lymphoproliferative syndrome (ALPS).

Clonal Anergy

Auto-reactive T cells when exposed to antigenic peptides on antigen presenting cells (APC) that do not possess the co-stimulatory molecules CD80 (B7-1) or CD86 (B7-2) become anergic (nonresponsive) to the antigen. Also, while activation of T cells through CD28 triggers IL-2 production, activation of CTLA4 leads to inhibition of IL-2 production and anergy. Also, B cells when exposed to large amounts of soluble antigen down-regulate their surface IgM and become anergic. These cells also up-regulate the Fas molecules on their surface. An interaction of these B cells with Fas-ligand bearing T cells results in their death via apoptosis.

Clonal Ignorance

T cells reactive to self-antigen not represented in the thymus will mature and migrate to the periphery, but they may never encounter the appropriate antigen because it is sequestered in inaccessible tissues.

Such cells may die out for lack of stimulus. Auto-reactive B cells, that escape deletion, may not find the antigen or the specific T-cell help and thus not be activated and die out.

Anti-idiotype Antibody

These are antibodies that are produced against the specific idiotypes of other antibodies. Anti-idiotypic antibodies are produced during the process of tolerization and have been demonstrated in tolerant animals. These antibodies may prevent the B cell receptor from interacting with the antigen.

Regulatory T Cells (Formerly Called Suppressor Cells)

Recently, a distinct population of T cells has been discovered called regulatory T cells. Regulatory T cells come in many flavors, but the most well characterized include those that express CD4+ and CD25+. Because activated normal CD4 T cells also express CD25, it was difficult to distinguish regulatory T cells and activated T cells. The latest research suggests that regulatory T cells are defined by expression of the forkhead family transcription factor Foxp3. Expression of Foxp3 is required for regulatory T cell development and function. The precise mechanism/s through which regulatory T cells suppress other T cell function is not clear. One of the mechanisms include the production of immunosuppressive cytokines such as TGF-β and IL-17, Genetic mutations in Foxp3 in humans leads to development of a severe and rapidly fatal auto-immune disorder known as Immune dysregulation, Polyendocrinopathy, Enteropathy, X-linked (IPEX) syndrome. This disease provides the most striking evidence that regulatory T cells play a critical role in preventing auto-immune disease.

Termination of Tolerance

Experimentally induced tolerance can be terminated by prolonged absence of exposure to the tolerogen, by treatments which severely damage the immune system (x-irradiation) or by immunization with cross reactive antigens. These observations are of significance in the conceptualization of auto-immune diseases.

Chapter

3

Immunoglobulins: Antigen-antibody Reactions

Nature of Antigen-antibody Reactions

Lock and Key Concept : The combining site of an antibody is located in the Fab portion of the molecule and is constructed from thehypervariable regions of the heavy and light chains. X-Ray crystallography studies of antigen-antibody interactions show that the antigenic determinant nestles in a cleft formed by the combining site of the antibody. Thus, our concept of antigen-antibody reactions is one of a key (*i.e.* the antigen) which fits into a lock (*i.e.* the antibody).

Non-covalent Bonds : The bonds that hold the antigen to the antibody combining site are all non-covalent in nature. These includehydrogen bonds, electrostatic bonds, Van der Waals forces and hydrophobic bonds. Multiple bonding between the antigen and the antibody ensures that the antigen will be bound tightly to the antibody.

Reversibility : Since antigen-antibody reactions occur via non-covalent bonds, they are by their nature reversible.

Affinity and Avidity

Affinity : Antibody affinity is the strength of the reaction between a single antigenic determinant and a single combining site on the antibody. It is the sum of the attractive and repulsive forces operating between the antigenic determinant and the combining site of the antibody. Affinity is the equilibrium constant that describes the antigen-antibody reaction. Most antibodies have a high affinity for their antigens.

Avidity : Avidity is a measure of the overall strength of binding of an antigen with many antigenic determinants and multivalent antibodies. Avidity is influenced by both the valence of the antibody and the valence of the antigen. Avidity is more than the sum of the individual affinities. To repeat, affinity refers to the strength of binding between a single antigenic determinant and an individual antibody combining site whereas avidity refers to the overall strength of binding between multivalent antigens and antibodies.

Specificity and Cross Reactivity

Specificity : Specificity refers to the ability of an individual antibody combining site to react with only one antigenic determinant or the ability of a population of antibody molecules to react with only one antigen. In general, there is a high degree of specificity in antigen-antibody reactions. Antibodies can distinguish differences in:

- The primary structure of an antigen
- Isomeric forms of an antigen
- Secondary and tertiary structure of an antigen.

Cross Reactivity : Cross reactivity refers to the ability of an individual antibody combining site to react with more than one antigenic determinant or the ability of a population of antibody molecules to react with more than one antigen. Cross reactions arise because the cross reacting antigen shares anepitope in common with the immunizing antigen or because it has an epitope which is structurally similar to one on the immunizing antigen (multispecificity).

Tests for Antigen-antibody Reactions

Factors Affecting Measurement of Antigen-antibody Reactions

The only way that one knows that an antigen-antibody reaction has occurred is to have some means of directly or indirectly detecting the complexes formed between the antigen and antibody. The ease with which one can detect antigen-antibody reactions will depend on a number of factors.

Affinity : The higher the affinity of the antibody for the antigen, the more stable will be the interaction. Thus, the ease with which one can detect the interaction is enhanced.

Avidity : Reactions between multivalent antigens and multivalent antibodies are more stable and thus easier to detect.

Antigen to antibody ratio : The ratio between the antigen and antibody influences the detection of antigen-antibody complexes because the size of the complexes formed is related to the concentration of the antigen and antibody.

Physical form of the antigen : The physical form of the antigen influences how one detects its reaction with an antibody. If the antigen is a particulate, one generally looks for agglutination of the antigen by the antibody. If the antigen is soluble one generally looks for the precipitation of the antigen after the production of large insoluble antigen-antibody complexes.

Agglutination Tests

Agglutination/Hemagglutination : When the antigen is particulate, the reaction of an antibody with the antigen can be detected by agglutination (clumping) of the antigen. The general term agglutinin is used to describe antibodies that agglutinate particulate antigens. When the antigen is an erythrocyte the term hemagglutination is used. All antibodies can theoretically agglutinate particulate antigens but IgM, due to its high valence, is particularly good agglutinin and one sometimes infers that an antibody may be of the IgM class if it is a good agglutinating antibody.

Qualitative agglutination test : Agglutination tests can be used in a qualitative manner to assay for the presence of an antigen or an antibody. The antibody is mixed with the particulate antigen and a positive test is indicated by the agglutination of the particulate antigen. For example, a patient's red blood cells can be mixed with antibody to a blood group antigen to determine a person's blood type. In a second example, a patient's serum is mixed with red blood cells of a known blood type to assay for the presence of antibodies to that blood type in the patient's serum.

Quantitative agglutination test : Agglutination tests can also be used to measure the level of antibodies to particulate antigens. In this test, serial dilutions are made of a sample to be tested for antibody and then a fixed number of red blood cells or bacteria or other such particulate antigen is added. Then the maximum dilution that gives agglutination is determined. The maximum dilution that gives visible agglutination is called the titter. The results are reported as the reciprocal of the maximal dilution that gives visible agglutination.

Prozone effect - Occasionally, it is observed that when the concentration of antibody is high (i.e. lower dilutions), there is no agglutination and then, as the sample is diluted, agglutination occurs. The lack of agglutination at high concentrations of antibodies is called the prozone effect. Lack of agglutination in the prozone is due to antibody excess resulting in very small complexes that do not clump to form visible agglutination.

Applications of agglutination tests;

i. Determination of blood types or antibodies to blood group antigens.

ii. To assess bacterial infections.

e.g. A rise in titter of an antibody to a particular bacterium indicates an infection with that bacterial type. N.B. a fourfold rise in titter is generally taken as a significant rise in antibody titter.

Practical considerations : Although the test is easy to perform, it is only semi-quantitative.

Passive hemagglutination : The agglutination test only works with particulate antigens. However, it is possible to coat erythrocytes with a soluble antigen (e.g. viral antigen, a polysaccharide or a hapten) and use the coated red blood cells in an agglutination test for antibody to the soluble antigen. This is called passive hemagglutination. The test is performed just like the agglutination test. Applications include detection of antibodies to soluble antigens and detection of antibodies to viral antigens.

Coomb's Test (Antiglobulin Test)

Direct Coomb's Test: When antibodies bind to erythrocytes, they do not always result in agglutination. This can result from the antigen/antibody ratio being in antigen excess or antibody excess or in some cases electrical charges on the red blood cells preventing the effective cross linking of the cells. These antibodies that bind to but do not cause agglutination of red blood cells are sometimes referred to as incomplete antibodies. In no way is this meant to indicate that the antibodies are different in their structure, although this was once thought to be the case. Rather, it is a functional definition only. In order to detect the presence of non-agglutinating antibodies on red blood cells, one simply adds a second antibody directed against the immunoglobulin (antibody) coating the red cells. This anti-immunoglobulin can now cross link the red blood cells and result in agglutination.

Indirect Coomb's Test : If it is necessary to know whether a serum sample has antibodies directed against a particular red blood cell and you want to be sure that you also detect potential non-agglutinating antibodies in the sample, an Indirect Coomb's test is performed. This test is done by incubating the red blood cells with the serum sample, washing out any unbound antibodies and then adding a second anti-immunoglobulin reagent to cross link the cells.

Applications

These include detection of anti-rhesus factor (Rh) antibodies. Antibodies to the Rh factor generally do not agglutinate red blood cells. Thus, red cells from Rh^+ children born to Rh^- mothers, who have anti-Rh antibodies, may be coated with these antibodies. To check for this, a direct Coombs test is performed. To see if the mother has anti-Rh antibodies in her serum an Indirect Coombs test is performed.

Hemagglutination Inhibition

The agglutination test can be modified to be used for the measurement of soluble antigens. This test is called hemagglutination inhibition. It is called hemagglutination inhibition because one measures the ability of soluble antigen to inhibit the agglutination of antigen-coated red blood cells by antibodies. In this test, a fixed amount of antibodies to the antigen in question is mixed with a fixed amount of red blood cells coated with the antigen. Also included in the mixture are different amounts of the sample to be analyzed for the presence of the antigen. If the sample contains the antigen, the soluble antigen will compete with the antigen coated on the red blood cells for binding to the antibodies, thereby inhibiting the agglutination of the red blood cells.

By serially diluting the sample, you can quantitate the amount of antigen in your unknown sample by its titter. This test is generally used to quantitate soluble antigens and is subject to the same practical considerations as the agglutination test.

Precipitation Tests

Radial Immunodiffusion (Mancini): In radial immunodiffusion antibody is incorporated into the agar gel as it is poured and different dilutions of the antigen are placed in holes punched into the agar. As the antigen diffuses into the gel, it reacts with the antibody and when the equivalence point is reached a ring of precipitation is formed.

The diameter of the ring is proportional to the log of the concentration of antigen since the amount of antibody is constant. Thus, by running different concentrations of a standard antigen one can generate a standard cure from which one can quantitate the amount of an antigen in an unknown sample. Thus, this is a quantitative test. If more than one ring appears in the test, more than one antigen/antibody reaction has occurred. This could be due to a mixture of antigens or antibodies. This test is commonly used in the clinical laboratory for the determination of immunoglobulin levels in patient samples.

Immunoelectrophoresis: In immunoelectrophoresis, a complex mixture of antigens is placed in a well punched out of an agar gel and the antigens are electrophoresed so that the antigen are separated according to their charge. After electrophoresis, a trough is cut in the gel and antibodies are added. As the antibodies diffuse into the agar, precipitin lines are produced in the equivalence zone when an antigen/antibody reaction occurs.

This tests is used for the qualitative analysis of complex mixtures of antigens, although a crude measure of quantity (thickness of the line) can be obtained. This test is commonly used for the analysis of components in a patient' serum. Serum is placed in the well and antibody to whole serum in the trough. By comparisons to normal serum, one can determine whether there are deficiencies on one or more serum components or whether there is an overabundance of some serum component (thickness of the line). This test can also be used to evaluate purity of isolated serum proteins.

Countercurrent Electrophoresis: In this test the antigen and antibody are placed in wells punched out of an agar gel and the antigen and antibody are electrophoresed into each other where they form a precipitation line. This test only works if conditions can be found where the antigen and antibody have opposite charges. This test is primarily qualitative, although from the thickness of the band you can get some measure of quantity. Its major advantage is its speed.

Radioimmunoassay (RIA)/Enzyme Linked Immunosorbent Assay (ELISA)

Radioimmunoassays (RIA) are assays that are based on the measurement of radioactivity associated with immune complexes. In any particular test, the label may be on either the antigen or the antibody. Enzyme Linked Immunosorbent Assays (ELISA) are those that are based on the measurement of an enzymatic reaction associated with immune complexes. In any particular assay, the enzyme may be linked to either the antigen or the antibody.

Competitive RIA/ELISA for AG Detection

The method and principle of RIA and ELISA for the measurement of antigen. By using known amounts of a standard unlabeled antigen, one can generate a standard curve relating radioactivity (cpm) (Enzyme) bound versus amount of antigen. From this standard curve, one can determine the amount of an antigen in an unknown sample.

The key to the assay is the separation of the immune complexes from the remainder of the components. This has been accomplished in many different ways and serves as the basis for the names given to the assay:

Precipitation with Ammonium Sulphate

Ammonium sulphate (33 - 50% final concentration) will precipitate immunoglobulins but not many antigens. Thus, this can be used to separate the immune complexes from free antigen. This has been called the Farr Technique

Anti-immunoglobulin Antibody

The addition of a second antibody directed against the first antibody can result in the precipitation of the immune complexes and thus the separation of the complexes from free antigen.

Immobilization of the Antibody

The antibody can be immobilized onto the surface of a plastic bead or coated onto the surface of a plastic plate and thus the immune complexes can easily be separated from the other components by simply washing the beads or plate. This is the most common method used today and is referred to as Solid phase RIA or ELISA. In the clinical laboratory, competitive RIA and ELISA are commonly used to quantitate serum proteins, hormones, drugs metabolites.

Non-competitive RIA/ELISA for AG or AB

Non-competitive RIA and ELISAs are also used for the measurement of antigens and antibodies. The amount of labeled second antibody bound is related to the amount of antibody in the unknown sample.

This assay is commonly employed for the measurement of antibodies of the IgE class directed against particular allergens by using a known allergen as antigen and anti-IgE antibodies as the labeled reagent. It is called the RAST test (radioallergosorbent test).

The bead is coated with antibody and is used to measure an unknown antigen. The amount of labeled second antibody that binds is proportional to the amount of antigen that bound to the first antibody.

Antibody Formation

General Characteristics of the Antibody Response

Self / Non-self Discrimination: One characteristic feature of the specific immune system is that it normally distinguishes between self and non-self and only reacts against non-self.

Memory: A second feature of the specific immune response is that it demonstrates memory. The immune system "remembers" if it has seen an antigen before and it reacts to secondary exposures to an antigen in a manner different than after a primary exposure. Generally only an exposure to the same antigen will illicit this memory response.

Specificity: A third characteristic feature of the specific immune system is that there is a high degree of specificity in its reactions. A response to a particular antigen is specific for that antigen or a few closely related antigens.

Kinetics of Antibody Responses to T-dependent Antigen

Primary (1°) Antibody Response

Inductive, Latent or Lag Phase: In this phase, the antigen is recognized as foreign and the cells begin to proliferate and differentiate in response to the antigen. The duration of this phase will vary depending on the antigen but it is usually 5 to 7 days.

Log or Exponential Phase

In this phase, the antibody concentration increases exponentially as the B cells that were stimulated by the antigen differentiate into plasma cells which secrete antibody.

Plateau or Steady-state Phase

In this phase, antibody synthesis is balanced by antibody decay so that there in no net increase in antibody concentration.

Decline or Decay Phase

In this phase, the rate of antibody degradation exceeds that of antibody synthesis and the level of antibody falls. Eventually the level of antibody may reach base line levels.

Secondary (2°), Memory or Anamnestic Response

Lag Phase: In a secondary response, there is a lag phase by it is normally shorter than that observed in a primary response.

Log phase: The log phase in a secondary response is more rapid and higher antibody levels are achieved.

Decline Phase: The decline phase is not as rapid and antibody may persist for months, years or even a lifetime.

Specificity of 1° and 2° Responses

Antibody elicited in response to an antigen is specific for that antigen, although it may also cross react with other antigens which are structurally similar to the eliciting antigen. In general secondary responses are only elicited by the same antigen used in the primary response. However, in some instances a closely related antigen may produce a secondary response, but this is a rare exception.

Qualitative Changes in Antibody During 1° and 2° Responses

Immunoglobulin Class Variation

In the primary response, the major class of antibody produced is IgM whereas in the secondary response it is IgG (or IgA or IgE). The antibodies that persist in the secondary response are the IgG antibodies.

Affinity

The affinity of the IgG antibody produced increases progressively during the response, particularly after low doses of antigen. This is referred to as affinity maturation. Affinity maturation is most pronounced after secondary challenge with antigen.

A second explanation for affinity maturation is that, after a class switch has occurred in the immune response, somatic mutations occur which fine tune the antibodies to be of higher affinity. There is experimental evidence for this mechanism, although it is not known how the somatic mutation mechanism is activated after exposure to antigen.

Avidity

As a consequence of increased affinity, the avidity of the antibodies increases during the response.

Cross-reactivity

As a result of the higher affinity later in the response, there is also an increase in detectible cross reactivity. An explanation for why increasing affinity results in an increase in detectible cross reactivity is illustrated by the following example.

	Early	***Late***
Immunizing Ag	10^{-6}	10^{-9}
	+	++
Cross reacting Ag	10^{-3}	10^{-6}
	-	+

If a minimum affinity of 10^{-6} is needed to detect a reaction, early in an immune response the reaction of a cross reacting antigen with an affinity of 10^{-3} will not be detected. However, late in a response when the affinities increase 1000 fold, the reaction with both the immunizing and cross reacting antigens will be detected.

Cellular Events During 1° and 2° Responses to T-dependent Antigen

Primary Response

Lag phase : Clones of T and B cells with the appropriate antigen receptors bind antigen, become activated and begin to proliferate. The expanded clones of B cells differentiate into plasma cells which begin to secrete antibody.

Log phase : The plasma cells initially secrete IgM antibody since the C_i heavy chain gene is closest to the rearranged VDJ gene. Eventually some B cells switch from making IgM to IgG, IgA or IgE. As more B cells proliferate and differentiate into antibody secreting cells the antibody concentration increases exponentially.

Stationary phase : As antigen is depleted, T and B cells are no longer activated. In addition, mechanisms which down regulate the immune response come into play.

Furthermore, plasma cells begin to die. When the rate of antibody synthesis equals the rate of antibody decay the stationary phase is reached.

Decline phase : When no new antibody is produced because the antigen is no longer present to activate T and B cells and the residual antibody slowly is degraded, the decay phase is reached.

Secondary Response

Not all of the T and B cells that are stimulated by antigen during primary challenge with antigen die. Some of them are long lived cells and constitute what is refer to as the memory cell pool. Both memory T cells and memory B cells are produced and memory T cells survive longer than memory B cells. Upon secondary challenge with antigen not only are virgin T and B cells activated, the memory cells are also activated and thus there is a shorter lag time in the secondary response. Since there is an expanded clone of cells being stimulated the rate of antibody production is also increased during the log phase of antibody production and higher levels are achieved. Also, since many if not all of the memory B cells will have switched to IgG (IgA or IgE) production, IgG is produced earlier in a secondary response. Furthermore since there is an expanded clone of memory T cells which can help B cells to switch to IgG (IgA or IgE) production, the predominant class of Ig produced after secondary challenge is IgG (IgA or IgE).

Ab Response to T-independent Antigen

Responses to T-independent antigen are characterized by the production of almost exclusively IgM antibody and no secondary response. Secondary exposure to the antigen results in another primary response to the antigen.

Class Switching

During an antibody response to a T-dependent antigen a switch occurs in the class of Ig produced from IgM to some other class (except IgD). Our understanding of the structure of the immunoglobulin genes, helps explain how class switching occurs.

During class switching another DNA rearrangement occurs between a switch site (S_μ) in the intron between the rearranged VDJ regions and the C_μ gene and another switch site before one of the other heavy chain constant region genes. The result of this recombination event is to bring the VDJ region close to one of the other constant region genes, thereby allowing expression of a new class of heavy chain. Since the same VDJ gene is brought near to a different C gene and since the antibody specificity is determined by the hypervariable regions within the V region, the antibody produced after the switch occurs will have the same specificity as before.

Cytokines secreted by T helper cells can cause the switch to certain isotypes.

Membrane and Secreted Immunoglobulin

The specificity of membrane immunoglobulin on a B cell and the Ig secreted by the plasma cell progeny of a B cell is the same. An understanding of how the specificity of membrane and secreted Ig from an individual B cell can be the same comes from an understanding of immunoglobulin genes.

There are two potential polyA sites in the immunoglobulin gene. One after the exon for the last heavy chain domain and the other after the exons that code for the trans- membrane domains. If the first polyA site is used, the pre-mRNA is processed to produce a secreted protein. If the second polyA site is used, the pre-mRNA is processed to produce a membrane form of the immunoglobulin. However, in all cases the same VDJ region is used and thus the specificity of the antibody remains the same. All C regions genes have these additional membrane pieces associated with them and thus after class switching other classes of immunoglobulins can be secreted or expressed on the surface of B cells.

Cells Involved in Immune Responses and Antigen Recognition

The immune system has developed to protect the host from pathogens and other foreign substances. Self/non-self discrimination is one of the hallmarks of the immune system. There are two main sites where pathogens may reside: extracellularly in tissue spaces or intracellularly within a host cell, and the immune system has different ways of dealing with pathogens at these sites. Although immune responses are tailored to the pathogen and to where the pathogen resides, most pathogens can elicit both an antibody and a cell-mediated response, both of which may contribute to ridding the host of the pathogen. However, for any particular pathogen an antibody or a cell-mediated response may be more important for defense against the pathogen.

Extracellular Pathogens

Antibodies are the primary defense against extracellular pathogens and they function in three major ways:

- Neutralization: By binding to the pathogen or foreign substance antibodies, can block the association of the pathogen with their targets. For example, antibodies to bacterial toxins can prevent the binding of the toxin to host cells thereby rendering the toxin ineffective. Similarly, antibody binding to a virus or bacterial pathogen can block the attachment of the pathogen to its target cell thereby preventing infection or colonization.

- Opsonization : Antibody binding to a pathogen or foreign substance can opsonize the material and facilitate its uptake and destruction by phagocytic cells. The Fc region of the antibody interacts with Fc receptors on phagocytic cells rendering the pathogen more readily phagocytosed.
- Complement activation : Activation of the complement cascade by antibody can result in lysis of certain bacteria and viruses. In addition, some components of the complement cascade (*e.g.* C3b) opsonize pathogens and facilitate their uptake via complement receptors on phagocytic cells.

Intracellular Pathogens

Because antibodies do not get into host cells, they are ineffective against intracellular pathogens. The immune system uses a different approach to deal with these kinds of pathogens. Cell-mediated responses are the primary defense against intracellular pathogens and the approach is different depending upon where the pathogen resides in the host cell (*i.e.*, in the cytosol or within vesicles). For example, most viruses and some bacteria reside in the cytoplasm of the host cell, however, some bacteria and parasites actually live within endosomes in the infected host cell. The primary defense against pathogens in the cytosol is the cytotoxic T lymphocyte (Tc or CTL). In contrast, the primary defense against a pathogen within vesicles is a subset of helper T lymphocytes (Th1).

- Cytotoxic T lymphocytes : CTLs are a subset of T lymphocytes that express a unique antigen on their surface called CD8. These cells recognize antigens from the pathogen that are displayed on the surface of the infected cell and kill the cell thereby preventing the spread of the infection to neighboring cells.
- CTLs kill by inducing apoptosis in the infected cell. Th cells are a subset of T cells that exprcss a unique antigen on their surface called CD4. A subpopulation of Th cells, Th1 cells, is the primary defense against intracellular pathogens that live within vesicles. Th1 cells recognize antigen from the pathogen that are expressed on the surface of infected cells and release cytokines that activate the infected cell. Once activated, the

infected cell can then kill the pathogen. For example, *Mycobacterium tuberculosis*, the causative agent of tuberculosis, infects macrophages but is not killed because it blocks the fusion of lysosomes with the endosomes in which it resides. Th1 cells that recognize *M. tuberculosis* antigens on the surface of an infected macrophage can secrete cytokines that activate macrophages. Once activated the lysosomes fuse with endosomes and the *M. tuberculosis* bacteria are killed.

Although immune responses are tailored to the pathogen and to where the pathogen resides, most pathogens can elicit both an antibody and a cell-mediated response, both of which may contribute to ridding the host of the pathogen. However, for any particular pathogen an antibody or a cell-mediated response may be more important for defense against the pathogen.

Cells of the Immune System

All cells of the immune system originate from a hematopoietic stem cell in the bone marrow, which gives rise to two major lineages, a myeloid progenitor cell and a lymphoid progenitor cell. These two progenitors give rise to the myeloid cells (monocytes, macrophages, dendritic cells, meagakaryocytes and granulocytes) and lymphoid cells (T cells, B cells and natural killer (NK) cells), respectively. Theses cells make up the cellular components of the innate (non-specific) and adaptive (specific) immune systems.

Cells of the Innate Immune System

Cells of the innate immune system include phagocytic cells (monocyte/macrophages and PMNs), NK cells, basophils, mast cells, eosinophiles and platelets. The roles of these cells have been discussed previously. The receptors of these cells are pattern recognition receptors (PRRs) that recognize broad molecular patterns found on pathogens (pathogen associated molecular patterns, PAMPS).

Cells that Link the Innate and Adaptive Immune Systems

A specialized subset of cells called antigen presenting cells (APCs) are a heterogenous population of leukocytes that play an important role in innate immunity and also act as a link to the adaptive immune system by participating in the activation of helper T cells (Th cells).

These cells include dendritic cells and macrophages. A characteristic feature of APCs is the expression of a cell surface molecule encoded by genes in the major histocompatibility complex, referred to as class II MHC molecules. B lymphocytes also express class II MHC molecules and they also function as APCs, although they are not considered as part of the innate immune system. In addition, certain other cells (*e.g.,* thymic epithelial cells) can express class II MHC molecules and can function as APCs.

Cells of the Adaptive Immune System

Cells that make up the adaptive (specific) immune system include the B and T lymphocytes. After exposure to antigen, B cells differentiate into plasma cells whose primary function is the production of antibodies. Similarly, T cells can differentiate into either T cytotoxic (Tc) or T helper (Th) cells of which there are two types Th1 and Th2 cells.

There are a number of cell surface markers that are used in clinical laboratories to distinguish B cells, T cells and their subpopulations.

Table : *Main distinguishing markers of T and B cells*

Marker	*B cells*	*Tc*	*Th*
CD3	-	+	+
CD4	-	-	+
CD8	-	+	-
CD19 and/or CD20	+	-	-
CD40	+	-	-
Ag receptor	BCR (surface Ig)	TCR	TCR

Specificity of the Adaptive Immune Response

Specificity on the adaptive immune response resides in the antigen receptors on T and B cells, the TCR and BCR, respectively. The TCR and BCR are similar in that each receptor is specific for one antigenic determinant but they differ in that BCRs are divalent while TCRs are monovalent. A consequence of this difference is that while B cells can have their antigen receptors cross-linked by antigen, TCRs cannot. This has implications as to how B and T cells can become activated.

Each B and T cells has a receptor that is unique for a particular antigenic determinant and there are a vast array of different antigen receptors on both B and T cells. The question of how these receptors are generated was the major focus of immunologists for many years. Two basic hypotheses were proposed to explain the generation of the receptors: the instructionist (template) hypothesis and the clonal selection hypothesis.

Instructionist Hypothesis

The instructionist hypothesis states that there is only one common receptor encoded in the germline and that different receptors are generated using the antigen as a template. Each antigen would cause the one common receptor to be folded to fit the antigen.

While this hypothesis was simple and very appealing, it was not consistent with what was known about protein folding (*i.e.* protein folding is dictated by the sequence of amino acids in the protein).

In addition this hypothesis did not account for self/non-self discrimination in the immune system. It could not explain why the one common receptor did not fold around self antigens.

Clonal Selection Hypothesis

The clonal selection hypothesis states that the germline encodes many different antigen receptors - one for each antigenic determinant to which an individual will be capable of mounting an immune response.

Antigen selects those clones of cells that have the appropriate receptor. The four basic principles of the clonal selection hypothesis are:

- Each lymphocyte bears a *single* type of receptor with a unique specificity.
- Interaction between a foreign molecule and a lymphocyte receptor capable of binding that molecule with a high affinity leads to lymphocyte activation.
- The differentiated effector cells derived from an activated lymphocyte will bear receptors of an identical specificity to those of the parental cell from which that lymphocyte was derived.
- Lymphocytes bearing receptors for self molecules are deleted at an early stage in lymphoid cell development and are therefore absent from the repertoire of mature lymphocytes.

The clonal selection hypothesis is now generally accepted as the correct hypothesis to explain how the adaptive immune system operates. It explains many of the features of the immune response:

1) the specificity of the response;
2) the signal required for activation of the response (*i.e.* antigen);
3) the lag in the adaptive immune response (time is required to activate cells and to expand the clones of cells); and
4) self/non-self discrimination.

Lymphocyte Recirculation

Since there are relatively few T or B lymphocytes with a receptor for any particular antigen (1/10,000 – 1/100,000), the chances for a successful encounter between an antigen and the appropriate lymphocyte are slim.

However, the chances for a successful encounter are greatly enhanced by the recirculation of lymphocytes through the secondary lymphoid organs.

Lymphocytes in the blood enter the lymph nodes and percolate through the lymph nodes. If they do not encounter an antigen in the lymph node, they leave via the lymphatics and return to the blood via the thoracic duct.

It is estimated that 1-2% of lymphocytes recirculate every hour. If the lymphocytes in the lymph nodes encounter an antigen, which has been transported to the lymph node via the lymphatics, the cells become activated, divide and differentiate to become a plasma cell, Th or Tc cell. After several days the effector cells can leave the lymph nodes via the lymphatics and return to the blood via the thoracic duct and then make their way to the infected tissue site.

Naive (virgin) lymphocytes enter the lymph nodes from the blood via High Endothelial Venules (HEVs) Homing receptors on the lymphocytes direct the cells to the HEVs.

In the lymph nodes, lymphocytes with the appropriate antigen receptor encounter antigen, which has been transported to the lymph nodes by dendritic cells or macrophages.

After activation the lymphocytes express new receptors that allow the cells to leave the lymph node and reenter the circulation.

Receptors on the activated lymphocytes recognize cell adhesion molecules expressed on endothelial cells near the site of an infection and chemokines produced at the infection site help attract the activated cells.

Immunity: Contrasts Between Non-specific and Specific

Non-specific (natural, native, innate);

- System in place prior to exposure to antigen
- Lacks discrimination among antigens
- Can be enhanced after exposure to antigen through effects of cytokines.

Specific (acquired, adaptive);

- Induced by antigen
- Enhanced by antigen
- Shows fine discrimination.

The hallmarks of the specific immune system are memory and specificity.

- The specific immune system "remembers" each encounter with a microbe or foreign antigen, so that subsequent encounters stimulate increasingly effective defense mechanisms.
- The specific immune response amplifies the protective mechanisms of non-specific immunity, directs or focuses these mechanisms to the site of antigen entry, and thus makes them better able to eliminate foreign antigens.

Cells of the Immune System

There are two main lineages that derive from the hemopoietic stem cell:

- The lymphoid lineage
  * T lymphocytes (T cells)
  * B lymphocytes (B cells)
  * Natural killer cells (NK cells).
- The myeloid lineage
  * Monocytes, macrophages
  * Langerhans cells, dendritic cells
  * Megakaryocytes
  * Granulocytes (eosinophils, neutrophils, basophils).

Clonal Selection

The four basic principles of the clonal selection hypothesis. Each lymphocyte bears a single type of receptor of a unique specificity. Interaction between a foreign molecule and a lymphocyte receptor capable of binding that molecule with high affinity leads to lymphocyte activation. The differentiated effector cells derived from an activated lymphocyte will bear receptors of an identical specificity to those of the parental cell from which that lymphocyte was derived. Lymphocytes bearing receptors specific for self molecules are deleted at an early stage in lymphoid cell development and are therefore absent from the repertoire of mature lymphocytes.

Major Histocompatibility Complex (Mhc) and T-cell Receptors - Role in Immune Responses

Teaching Objectives

To give an overview of the role of the major histocompatibility complex in immune responses.

To describe the structure and function of class I and class II MHC molecules.

To discuss the nature of polymorphisims in class I and class II MHC molecules.

To describe the structure of the T cell receptor for antigen

To discuss the genetic basis for the generation of diversity in the TCR.

To discuss the role of the CD3 complex and co-stimulatory molecules.

To describe the nature of the immunological synapse.

To discuss the requirements for T cell active.

Historical Overview

Cell-cell interactions of the adaptive immune response are critically important in protection from pathogens. These interactions are orchestrated by the immunological synapse whose primary components are the T cell antigen receptor (TCR) and the Major histocompatibility complex (MHC) molecule. The major function of the TCR is to recognize antigen in the correct context of MHC and to transmit an excitatory signal to the interior of the cell. Since binding of peptide within the MHC is not covalent, there are many factors while help stabilize the immunological synapse.

Gene products encoded in the MHC were first identified as being important in rejection of transplanted tissues. Furthermore, genes in the MHC were found to be highly polymorphic (i.e. in the population there were many different allelic forms of the genes). Studies with inbred strains of mice showed that genes in the MHC were also involved in controlling both humoral and cell-mediated immune responses. For example, some strains of mice could respond to a particular antigen but other strains could not and these strains differed only in one or more of the genes in the MHC. Subsequent studies showed that there were two kinds of molecules encoded by the MHC – Class I molecules and class II molecules which are recognized by different classes of T cells. Class I molecules were found on all nucleated cells (not red blood cells) whereas class II molecules were found only on antigen presenting cells, (APCs) which included dendritic cells, macrophages, B cells and a few other types.

It was not until the discovery of how the TCR recognizes antigen that the role of MHC genes in immune responses was understood. The TCR was shown to recognize antigenic peptides in association with MHC molecules. T cells recognize portions of protein antigens that are bound non-covalently to MHC gene products. Cytotoxic T cells (Tc) recognize peptides bound to class I MHC molecules and helper T cells (Th) recognize peptides bound to class II MHC molecules.

The three dimensional structures of MHC molecules and the TCR have been determined by X-ray crystallography so that a clear picture of how the TCR, MHC gene products and antigen interact has emerged.

Structure of Class I MHC Molecules

The Molecule: Class I MHC molecules are composed of two polypeptide chains, a long *a* chain and a short *a* chain called *a*2-microglobulin. The *a* chain has four regions.

- A cytoplasmic region, containing sites for phosphoylation and binding to cytoskeletal elements.
- A transmembrane region containing hydrophic amino acids by which the molecule is anchored in the cell membrane.
- A highly conserved *a*3 immunoglubilin-like domain to which CD8 binds.
- A highly polymorphic peptide binding region formed from the *a*1 and *a*2 domains. The *a*2- microglobulin associates with the *a* chain and helps maintain the proper conformation of the molecule.

The Antigen-binding Groove: An analysis of which part of the class I MHC molecules is most variable demonstrates that variability is most pronounced in the *a*1 and *a*2 domains, which comprise the peptide binding region. The structure of the peptide binding groove, revealed by X-ray crystallography, shows that the groove is composed of two *a* helices forming a wall on each side and eight â-pleated sheets forming a floor.

The peptide is bound in the groove and the residues that line the groove make contact with the peptide. These are the residues that are the most polymorphic.

The groove will accommodate peptides of approximately 8-10 amino acids long. Whether a particular peptide will bind to the groove will depend on the amino acids that line the groove. Because class I molecules are polymorphic, different class I molecules will bind different peptides. Each class I molecule will bind only certain peptides and will have a set of criteria that a peptide must have in order to bind to the groove.

As long as these two conditions are met a peptide will bind, regardless of what the other amino acids are. Similarly a different class I molecule will bind any peptide that has a tyrosine (Y) as the second amino acid from the amino-terminal end and either a valine (V), isoleucine (I) or leucine (L) at the carboxy-terminal end. Thus, for every class I molecule, there are certain amino acids that must be a particular location in the peptide before it will bind to the MHC molecule. These sites in the peptide are referred to as the "anchor sites". The ends of the peptide are buried within the closed ends of the class I binding groove while the center bulges out for presentation to the TCR.

Within the MHC there are 6 genes that encode class I molecules HLA-A, HLA –B, HLA-C, HLA-E, HLA-F and HLA-G. Among these HLA-A, HLA –B, and HLA-C are the most important and are most polymorphic.

Table: *Polymorphism of class I MHC genes*

Locus	***Number of alleles (allotypes)***
HLA-A	218
HLA-B	439
HLA-C	96
HLA-E, HLA-F and HLA-G	Relatively few alleles

Structure of Class II MHC Molecules

The Molecule: Class II MHC molecules are composed of two polypeptide chains an α and a β chain of approximately equal length. Both chains have four regions:

- A cytoplasmic region containing sites for phosphoylation and binding to cytoskeletal elements
- A transmembrane region containing hydrophic amino acids by which the molecule is anchored in the cell membrane

- A highly conserved α2 domain and a highly conserved α2 domain to which CD4 binds
- A highly polymorphic peptide binding region formed from the α1 and α1 domains.

The Antigen-binding Groove

As with Class I MHC molecules, an analysis of which part of the class II MHC molecule is most variable demonstrates that variability is most pronounced in the α1 and β1 domains, which comprise the peptide binding region. The structure of the peptide binding groove, revealed by X-ray crystallography, shows that, like class I MHC molecules, the groove is composed of two α helices forming a wall on each side and eight α-pleated sheets forming a floor.

Both the α1 and β1 chain contribute to the peptide binding groove. The peptide is bound in the groove and the residues that line the groove make contact with the peptide. These are the residues that are the most polymorphic. The groove of Class II molecules is open at one end so that the groove can accommodate longer peptides of approximately 13-25 amino acids long with some of the amino acids located outside of the groove.

Whether a particular peptide will bind to the groove will depend on the amino acids that line the groove. Because class II molecules are polymorphic, different class II molecules will bind different peptides. Like class I molecules, each class II molecule will bind only certain peptides and will have a set of criteria that a peptide must have in order to bind to the groove (i.e. "anchor sites").

Within the MHC there are 5 loci that encode class II molecules, each of which contains a gene for an α chain and at least one gene for a α chain. The loci are designated as HLA-DP, HLA –DQ, HLA-DR, HLA-DM, and HLA-DO. Among these, HLA-DP, HLA –DQ, and HLA-DR are the most important and are most polymorphic.

Important Aspects of MHC

- Although there is a high degree of polymorphism for a species, an individual has maximum of six different class I MHC products and only slightly more class II MHC products (considering only the major loci).
- Each MHC molecule has only one binding site. The different peptides a given MHC molecule can bind all bind to the same site, but only one at a time.

- Because each MHC molecule can bind many different peptides, binding is termed degenerate.
- MHC polymorphism is determined only in the germline. There are no recombinational mechanisms for generating diversity.
- MHC molecules are membrane-bound; recognition by T cells requires cell-cell contact.
- Alleles for MHC genes are co-dominant. Each MHC gene product is expressed on the cell surface of an individual nucleated cell.
- A peptide must associate with a given MHC of that individual, otherwise no immune response can occur. That is one level of control.
- Mature T cells must have a T cell receptor that recognizes the peptide associated with MHC. This is the second level of control.
- Cytokines (especially interferon-γ) increase level of expression of MHC.
- Peptides from the cytosol associate with class I MHC and are recognized by Tc cells. Peptides from within vesicles associate with class II MHC and are recognized by Th cells.
- Polymorphism in MHC is important for survival of the species.

How do Peptides Get into the MHC Groove?

Peptides from the cytosol associate with class I MHC and are recognized by CTL cells. The peptides enter the endoplasmic reticulum and bind in the MHC class I groove. This complex is then exported to the cell surface through the Golgi. MHC class II molecules are formed with an invariant (Ii) chain as a place holder while in the ER and Golgi. The Ii chain is cleaved and removed once the complex is in a vesicle. Peptides from within the vesicle associate with class II MHC and are then exported to the cell surface where they are recognized by Th cells.

Table: *Polymorphism of class II MHC genes*

Locus	***Number of alleles (allotypes)***
HLA-DPA	12
HLA-DPB	88
HLA-DQA	17
HLA-DQB	42

Contd...

Locus	*Number of alleles (allotypes)*
HLA-DRA	2
HLA-DRB1	269
HLA-DRB3	30
HLA-DRB4	7
HLA-DRB5	12
HLA-DM and HLA-DO	Relatively few alleles

The Role of TCR in the Immune Response

The TCR is a surface molecule found on T cells that recognizes antigen presented in the correct MHC context. The TCR is similar to immunoglobulin and is part of the immunoglobulin superfamily. There are two types of TCRs, the predominant αβ which is commonly found in lymphoid tissues, and the γδ which is found at mucosal surfaces.

Structure of the T Cell Receptor (TCR)

The TCR is a heterodimer composed of one α and one β chain of approximately equal length. Each chain has a short cytoplasmic tail but it is to small to be able to transduce an activation signal to the cell. Both chains have a transmembrane region comprised of hydrophobic amino acids by which the molecule is anchored in the cell membrane. Both chains have a constant region and a variable region similar to the immunoglobulin chains. The variable region of both chains contains hypervariable regions that determine the specificity for antigen. Each T cell bears a TCR of only one specificity (*i.e.* there is allelic exclusion).

The Genetic Basis for Receptor Generation

The genetic basis for the generation of the vast array of antigen receptors on B cells has been discussed previously. The generation of a vast array of TCRs is accomplished by similar mechanism. The germline genes for the TCR α genes are composed of V, D and J gene segments that rearrange during T cell development to produce many different TCR β chains. The germline genes for the TCR α genes are composed of V and J gene segments which rearrange to produce α chains. The specificity of the TCR is determined by the combination of α and β chains.

There is a small population of T cells that express TCRs that have γ and δ chains instead of α and β chains. These gamma/delta T cells predominate in the mucosal epithelium and have a repertoire biased toward certain bacterial and viral antigens. The genes for the δ chains have V, D and J gene segments whereas the genes for the β chains have only V and J gene segments but the repertoire is considerably smaller that than that of the alpha/beta T cells. The gamma/delta T cells recognize antigen in an MHC-independent manner unlike the alpha/beta T cells.

Important Aspects of the TCR

- Each T cell bears a TCR of only one specificity (i.e. there is allelic exclusion).
- The αβ TCR recognizes antigen only in the context of cell-cell interaction and in the correct MHC.
- The αδ TCR recognizes antigen in an MHC-independent manner in response to certain viral and bacterial antigen.

TCR and CD3 Complex

The TCR is closely associated with a group of 5 proteins collectively called the CD3 complex. The CD3 complex is composed of one γ, one δ, two ε and 2 ξ chains. All of the proteins of the CD3 complex are invariant and they do not contribute to the specificity in any way. The CD 3 complex is necessary for cell surface expression of the TCR during T cell development. In addition, the CD3 complex transduces activation signals to the cell following antigen interaction with the TCR of co-stimulatory molcules in the absence of TCR engagement results in no response

***Table** : Comparison of the Major Properties of Immunoglobulin (IG) And T-cell Receptor (TCR) Genes and Proteins*

Genes		
Properties	Ig	TCR
Many VDJs, Few C's	Yes	Yes
VDJ Rearrangement	Yes	Yes
V pairs form antigen-recognition site	Yes	Yes
Somatic hypermutation	Yes	No
Proteins		
Transmembrane forms	Yes	Yes
Secreted forms	Yes	No
Isotypes with distinct functions	Yes	No
Valency	2	1

Adapted from Janeway and Travers, Immunobiology

The "Immunological Synapse"

The interaction between the TCR and MHC molecules are not very strong. Accessory molecules are necessary to help stabilize the interaction. These include:

- CD4 binding to Class II MCH, which ensures that Th cells only interact with APCs
- CD8 binding to class I MHC, which ensures that Tc cells can interact with target cells
- CD2binding to LFA-3
- LFA-1 binding to ICAM-1

The accessory molecules are invariant and do not contribute to the specificity of the interaction, which is solely determined by the TCR. The expression of accessory molecules can be increased in response to cytokine, which is one way that cytokines can modulate immune responses.

In addition to accessory molecules which help stabilize the interaction between the TCR and antigen in association with MHC molecules, other molecules are also needed for T cell activation. Two signals are required for T cell activation – one is the engagement of the TCR with Ag/MHC and the other signal comes from the engagement of co-stimulatory molecules with their ligands.

One of the most important (but not the only) co-stimulatory molecule is CD28 on T cells which must interact with B7-1 (CD80) or B7-2 (CD81) on APCs . Like accessory molecules the co-stimulatory molecules are invariant and do not contribute to the specificity of the interaction. The multiple interactions of TCR with Ag/MHC and the accessory and co-stimulatory molecules with their ligands have been termed the "immunological synapse."

Not only is co-stimulation necessary for T cell activation, a lack of co-stimulation may result in anergy (i.e., inability to respond to antigen) or down-regulation of the response. Engagement of the TCR with Ag/MHC but no co-simulation results in anergy. Engagement of only the co-stimulatory molecule has no effect. Engagement of TCR with Ag/MHC and co-stimulatory molecules with their ligand results in activation.

Engagement of the TCR with Ag/MHC and engagement of B7 ligand with CTLA-4, molecules similar to CD28, results in down-regulation of the response. CTLA-4/B7 interaction sends an inhibitory signal to the T cell rather than an activating signal. This is one of the ways that immune responses are regulated. CTLA-4 is expressed on T cells later in an immune response and this helps to turn off the response.

Key Steps in T Cell Activation

- APC must process and present peptides to T cells
- T cells must receive a co-stimulatory signal - usually from CD28/B7
- Accessory adhesion molecules must help to stabilize the binding of T cells and APC. (CD4/class II MHC, CD8/classs I MHC, LFA-1/ICAM-1 and CD2/LFA-3)
- Signals from cell surface must be transmitted to the nucleus via second messengers
- Cytokines, including IL-2, must help drive cell division.

Table : *Important Accessory Molecules*

T cell molecule	*Ligand on second cell*
CD4 on helper T cells	class II MHC molecules
CD8 on cytotoxic T cells	class I MHC molecules
LFA-2 (CD2)	LFA-3
LFA-1	ICAM-1, ICAM-2

LFA = Leukocyte Function-associated Antigen

ICAM = Intercellular Adhesion Molecule

Response to Antigen: Processing and Presentation MHC Restriction and Role of the Thymus

Comparison of BCR and TCR : B cells and T cells recognize different substances as antigens and in a different form. The B cell uses cell surface-bound immunoglobulin as a receptor and the specificity of that receptor is the same as the immunoglobulin that it is able to secrete after activation. B cells recognize the following antigens in soluble form:

- Proteins (both conformational determinants and determinants exposed by denaturation or proteolysis)
- Nucleic acids
- Polysaccharides
- Some lipids
- Small chemicals (haptens).

In contrast, the overwhelming majority of antigens for T cells are proteins, and these must be fragmented and recognized in association with MHC products expressed on the surface of nucleated cells, not in a soluble form. T cells are grouped functionally according to the class of MHC molecules that associate with the peptide fragments of the protein: helper T cells recognize only those peptides associated with class II MHC molecules, and cytotoxic T cells recognize only those peptides associated with class I MHC molecules.

Antigen Processing and Presentation

Antigen processing and presentation are processes that occur within a cell that result in fragmentation (proteolysis) of proteins, association of the fragments with MHC molecules, and expression of the peptide-MHC molecules at the cell surface where they can be recognized by the T cell receptor on a T cell. However, the path leading to the association of protein fragments with MHC molecules differs for class I and class II MHC. MHC class I molecules present degradation products derived from intracellular (endogenous) proteins in the cytosol. MHC class II molecules present fragments derived from extracellular (exogenous) proteins that are located in an intracellular compartment.

Antigen Processing and Presentation in Cells Expressing Class I MHC

Proteins are fragmented in the cytosol by proteosomes (a complex of proteins having proteolytic activity) or by other proteases. The fragments are then transported across the membrane of the endoplasmic reticulum by transporter proteins. (The transporter proteins and some components of the proteosome have their genes in the MHC complex). Synthesis and assembly of class I heavy chain and $beta_2$ microglobulin occurs in the endoplasmic reticulum. Within the endoplasmic reticulum, the MHC class I heavy chain, $beta_2$microglobulin and peptide form a stable complex that is transported to the cell surface.

Antigen Processing and Presentation in Cells Expressing Class II MHC

Whereas all nucleated cells express class I MHC, only a limited group of cells express class II MHC, which includes the antigen presenting cells (APC). The principal APC are macrophages, dendritic cells (Langerhans cells), and B cells, and the expression of class II MHC molecules is either constitutive or inducible, especially by interferon-gamma in the case of macrophages.

Exogenous proteins taken in by endocytosis are fragmented by proteases in anendosome. The alpha and beta chains of MHC class II, along with an invariant chain, are synthesized, assembled in the endoplasmic reticulum, and transported through the Golgi and trans-Golgi apparatus to reach the endosome, where the invariant chain is digested, and the peptide fragments from the exogenous protein are able to associate with the class II MHC molecules, which are finally transported to the cell surface.

Web Resources

Important aspects of antigen processing and presentation;

- One way of rationalizing the development of two different pathways is that each ultimately stimulates the population of T cells that is most effective in eliminating that type of antigen.
- Viruses replicate within nucleated cells in the cytosol and produce endogenous antigens that can associate with class I MHC. By killing these infected cells, cytolytic T cells help to control the spread of the virus.
- Bacteria mainly reside and replicate extracellularly. By being taken up and fragmented inside cells as exogenous antigens that can associate with class II MHC molecules, helper Th2 T cells can be activated to assist B cells to make antibody against bacteria, which limits the growth of these organisms.
- Some bacteria grow intracellularly inside the vesicles of cells like macrophages. Inflammatory Th1 T cells help to activate macrophages to kill the intracellular bacteria.
- Fragments of self, as well as non-self, proteins associate with MHC molecules of both classes and are expressed at the cell surface.
- Which protein fragments bind is a function of the chemical nature of the groove for that specific MHC molecule.

Self MHC Restriction

In order for a T cell to recognize and respond to a foreign protein antigen, it must recognize the MHC on the presenting cell as self MHC.

This is termed self MHC restriction. Helper T cells recognize antigen in context of class II self MHC. Cytolytic T cells recognize antigen in context of class I self MHC. The process whereby T cells become restricted to recognizing self MHC molecules occurs in the thymus. The experimental systems demonstrating self MHC restriction for APC-helper T cell interactions and for class I MHC-cytotoxic T cell interactions.

Antigen Presenting Cells

The three main types of antigen presenting cells are dendritic cells, macrophages and B cells, although other cells, that express class II MHC molecules, (*e.g.*, thymic epithelial cells) can act as antigen presenting cells in some cases. Dendritic cells, which are found in skin and other tissues, ingest antigens by pinocytosis and transport antigens to the lymph nodes and spleen. In the lymph nodes and spleen they are found predominantly in the T cells areas. Dendritic cells are the most effective antigen presenting cells and can present antigens to naïve (virgin) T cells.

Furthermore, they can present internalized antigens in association with either class I or class II MHC molecules (cross presentation), although the predominant pathway for internalized antigen is the class II pathway. The second type of antigen presenting cell is the macrophage. These cells ingest antigen by phagocytosis or pinocytosis. Macrophages are not as effective in presenting antigen to naïve T cells but they are very good in activating memory T cells. The third type of antigen presenting cell is the B cell. These cells bind antigen via their surface immunoglobulin and ingest antigens by pinocytosis. Like macrophages these cells are not as effective as dendritic cells in presenting antigen to naïve T cells. B cells are very effective in presenting antigen to memory T cells, especially when the antigen concentration is low because surface immunoglobulin on the B cells binds antigen with a high affinity.

Presentation of Superantigens

Superantigens are antigens that can polyclonally activate T cells to produce large quantities of cytokines that can have pathological effects. These antigens must be presented to T cells in association with class II MHC molecules but the antigen does not need to be processed. In the case of a superantigen, the intact protein binds to class II MHC molecules and to one or more V_β regions of the TCR. The antigen is not bound to the peptide binding groove of the MHC molecule or to the antigen binding site of the TCR. Thus, any T cell that uses a particular V in its TCR will be activated by a superantigen, resulting in the activation of a large numbers of T cells. Each superantigen will bind to a different set of V_β regions.

Thymic Education

Both Th and Tc cells are self-MHC restricted. In addition, T cells do not normally recognize self antigens. How are self MHC restricted T cells generated and why are self reacting T cells not produced? Random VDJ rearrangements in T cells would be expected to generate some T cells that can recognize non-self MHC and some T cells that can recognize self antigens. It is the role of the thymus to ensure that the only T cells that get to the periphery are self-MHC restricted and unable to react with self antigen. Functional T cells in the periphery have to recognize foreign antigens associated with self MHC, because APC or target cells present foreign antigen associated with self MHC. However, an individual does not need functional T cells in the periphery that recognize antigen (self or foreign) associated with foreign MHC. An individual especially does not want functional T cells in the periphery that can recognize self antigens associated with self MHC because they could lead to damage of healthy, normal tissues.

As a result of random VDJ recombination events occurring in immature T cells within the thymus, TCRs of all specificities are produced. Processes in the thymus determine which TCR specificities are retained. First, T cells with the ability to bind to self MHC molecules expressed by cortical thymic epithelial cells are retained. This is known as positive selection. Those that do not bind, undergo apoptosis. Thus, T cells having a TCR that recognizes self MHC survive. Next, T cells with the ability to bind to self MHC molecules associated with self molecules expressed by thymic epithelial cells, dendritic cells and macrophages are killed. This is known as negative selection. Those that do not bind are retained. As a result of these two steps, T cells having a TCR that recognizes self MHC and foreign antigen survive. Each T cell that survives positive and negative selection in the thymus and is released into the periphery retains its specific T cell receptor.

While positive and negative selection is occurring in the thymus the immature T cells are also expressing CD4 or CD8 antigens on their surface. Initially the pre-T cell that enters the thymus is CD4-CD8-. In the thymus it becomes CD4+CD8+ and as positive and negative selection proceeds a cell becomes either a CD4+ or CD8+ cell. The commitment to become either a CD4+ or CD8+ cells depends on which class of MHC molecule the cell encounters. If a CD4+CD8+ cell is presented with a class I molecule it will down regulate CD4 and become a CD8+ cell. If a cell is presented with a class II MHC molecule it will down regulate CD8 and become a CD4+ cell.

Negative Selection in the Periphery

Positive and negative selection in the thymus is not a 100% efficient process. In addition, not all self antigens may be expressed in the thymus. Thus some self reactive T cells may get to the periphery. Thus, there are additional mechanisms that are designed to eliminate self reactive T cells in the periphery.

B Cell Selection

Since B cells are not MHC-restricted there is no need for positive selection of B cells. However, negative selection (i.e., elimination of self-reactive clones) of B cells is required. This occurs during B cell development in the bone marrow. However, negative selection of B cells is not a critical as for T cells since, in most instances, B cells require T cell help in order to become activated. Thus, if a self reactive B cell does get to the periphery it will not be activated due to lack of T cell help.

Cell-mediated Immunity: Cell-cell Interactions in Specific Immune Responses

Central Role of TH Cells in Immune Responses

After Th cells recognize specific antigen presented by an antigen-presenting cell (APC), they can initiate several key immune processes. These include: 1) selection of appropriate effector mechanisms (e.g., B cell activation or Tc generation); 2) induction of proliferation of appropriate effector cells and 3) enhancement of the functional activities of other cells (e.g., granulocytes, macrophages, NK cells).

There are four subpopulations of Th cells: Th0, Th1, Th2 and Th17 cells. When naïve Th0 cells encounter antigen in secondary lymphoid tissues, they are capable of differentiating into inflammatory Th1 cells, helper Th2 cells or pathogenic T17 cells, which are distinguished by the cytokines they produce. Whether a Th0 cells becomes a Th1, a Th2 or a T17 cell depends upon the cytokines in the environment, which is influenced by antigen. For example some antigens stimulate IL-4 production which favours the generation of Th2 cells while other antigens stimulate IL-16, production, which favours the generation of Th1 cells. Th1, Th2 and Th17 cells affect different cells and influence the type of an immune response.

Cytokines produced by Th1 cells activate macrophages and participate in the generation of cytoxic lymphocytes (CTL), resulting in a cell-mediated immune response. In contrast cytokines produced by Th2 cells help to activate B cells, resulting in antibody production.

In a relatively recent discovery, Th17 cells (designated as such by their production of IL-17) differentiate (in humans) in response to IL-1, IL-6, and IL-6, TGF-β is important for Th17 differentiation in mice, but not in humans. IL-6, enhances the severity of some autoimmune diseases including multiple sclerosis, inflammatory bowel disease, and rheumatoid arthritis.

Equally important, each subpopulation can exert inhibitory influences on the other. IFN-γ produced by Th1 cells inhibits proliferation of Th2 cells and differentiation of Th17 cells and IL-6, produced by Th2 cells inhibits production of IFN-β by Th1 cells. In addition, although not shown, IL-4 inhibits production of Th1 cells and differentiation of Th17 cells. Thus, the immune response is directed to the type of response that is required to deal with the pathogen encountered – cell-mediated responses for intracellular pathogens or antibody responses for extracellular pathogens.

Cell-cell Interactions in Antibody Responses to Exogenous T-dependent Antigens

Hapten-carrier Model

Historically one of the major findings in immunology was that both T cells and B cells were required for antibody production to a complex protein. A major contribution to our understanding of this process came from studies on the formation of anti-hapten antibodies. Studies with hapten-carrier conjugates established that:

- Th2 cells recognized the carrier determinants and B cells recognized haptenic determinants
- Interactions between hapten-specific B cells and carrier-specific Th cells was self MHC restricted
- B cells can function both in antigen recognition and in antigen presentation.

B cells occupy a unique position in immune responses because they express immunoglobulin and class II MHC molecules on their cell surface. They therefore are capable of producing antibody having the same specificity as that expressed by their immunoglobulin receptor; in addition they can function as an antigen presenting cell. In terms of the hapten-carrier conjugate model, the mechanism is thought to be the following:

The hapten is recognized by the immunoglobulin receptor, the hapten-carrier is brought into the B cell, processed, and peptide fragments of the carrier protein are presented to a helper T cell. Activation of the T cell results in the production of cytokines that enable the hapten-specific B cell to become activated to produce soluble anti-hapten antibodies.

Note that there are multiple signals delivered to the B cells in this model of Th2 cell-B cell interaction. As was the case for activation of T cells where the signal derived from the TCR recognition of a peptide-MHC molecule was by itself insufficient for T cell activation, so too for the B cell. Binding of an antigen to the immunoglobulin receptor delivers one signal to the B cell, but that is insufficient. Second signals delivered by co-stimulatory molecules are required; the most important of these is CD40L on the T cell that binds to CD40 on the B cell to initiate delivery of a second signal.

Cell-cell Interactions in the Primary Antibody Response

B cells are not the best antigen presenting cell in a primary antibody response; dendritic cells or macrophages are more efficient. Nevertheless, with some minor modifications the hapten-carrier model of cell-cell interactions described above also applies to interactions in a primary antibody response.

In a primary response the Th2 cell first encounters antigen presented by dendritic cells or macrophages. The “primed” Th2 cell can then interact with B cells that have encountered antigen and are presenting antigenic peptides in association with class II MHC molecules.

The B cells still require two signals for activation – one signal is the binding of antigen to the surface immunoglobulin and the second signal comes from CD40/CD40 ligand engagement during Th2/B cell-cell interaction. In addition, cytokines produced by the Th2 cells help B cells proliferate and differentiate into antibody secreting plasma cells.

Cell-cell Interactions in the Secondary Antibody Responses

As a consequence of a primary response, many memory T and B cells are produced. Memory B cells have a high affinity immunoglobulin receptor (due to affinity maturation), which allows them to bind and present antigen at much lower concentrations than that required for macrophages or dendritic cells. In addition, memory T cells are more easily activated than naïve T cells.

Thus, B/Th cell interactions are sufficient to generate secondary antibody responses. It is not necessary (although it can occur) to "prime" memory Th cells with antigen presented by dendritic cells or macrophages.

Cytokines and Class Switching

Cytokines produced by activated Th2 cells not only stimulate proliferation and differentiation of B cells, they also help regulate the class of antibody produced.

Different cytokines influence the switch to different classes of antibodies with different effort functions. In this way the antibody response is tailored to suit the pathogen encountered (e.g. IgE antibodies for parasitic worm infections).

Cell-cell Interactions in Antibody Responses to Exogenous T-independent Antigens

Antibody responses to T-independent antigens do not require cell-cell interactions. The polymeric nature of these antigens allows cross-linking of antigen receptors on B cells resulting in activation. No secondary responses, affinity maturation or class switching occurs. Responses to T-independent antigens are due to the activation of a subpopulation of B cells called CD5+ B cells (also called B1 cells), which distinguishes them from conventional B cells that are CD5- (also called B2 cells).

CD5+ (B1) Cells

CD5+ cells are the first B cells to appear in ontogeny. They express surface IgM but little or no IgD and they produce primarily IgM antibodies from minimally somatically mutated germ line genes. Antibodies produced by these cells are of low affinity and are often polyreactive (bind multiple antigens).

Most of the IgM in serum is derived from CD5+ B cells. CD5+ B cells do not give rise to memory cells. An important characteristic of these cells is that they are self-renewing, unlike conventional B cells which must be replaced from the bone marrow. CD5+ B cells are found in peripheral tissues and are the predominant B cell in the peritoneal cavity. B1 cells are a major defense against many bacterial pathogens that characteristically have polysaccharides in their cell walls. The importance of these cells in immunity is illustrated by the fact that many individuals with T cell defects are still able to resist many bacterial pathogens.

Cell-cell Interactions in Cell-mediated Immunity - Generation of TC Cells in Response to Endogenous Antigens in the Cytosol

Cytotoxic T lymphocytes are not fully mature when they exit the thymus.

They have a functional TCR that recognizes antigen, but they cannot lyse a target cell. They must differentiate into fully functional effector Tc cells.

Cytotoxic cells differentiate from a "pre-CTL" in response to two signals:

- Specific antigen in the context of class I MHC, on a stimulator cell
- Cytokines produced by Th1 cells, especially IL-2, and IFN-gamma.

Features of CTL-mediated Lysis

- CTL killing is antigen-specific. To be killed by a CTL, the target cell must bear the same class I MHC-associated antigen that triggered pre-CTL differentiation.
- apoptosis.
    - o Fas- and TNF-mediated killing.

      Once generated CTLs express Fas ligand on their surface, which binds to Fas receptors on target cells. In addition, TNF-α secreted by CTLs can bind to TNF receptors on target cells. The Fas and TNF receptors are a closely related family of receptors, which when they encounter their ligands, for trimers of the receptors. These receptors also contain death domains in the cytoplasmic portion of the receptor, which after trimerization can activate caspases that induce apoptosis in the target cell.
    - o Granule-mediated killing

      Fully differentiated CTLs have numerous granules that contain perforin and granzymes. Upon contact with target cells, perforin is released and it polymerizes to form channels in the target cell membrane. Granzymes, which are serine proteases, enter the target cell through the channels and activate caspases and nucleases in the target cell resulting in apoptosis.

Cell-cell Interactions in Cell-mediated Immunity - Activation of Macrophages in Response to Endogenous Antigens in Vesicles

Macrophages play a central role in the immune system. Macrophages are involved in:

- Initial defense as part of the innate immune system
- Antigen presentation to Th cells
- Various effector functions (*e.g.*, cytokine production, bactericidal and tumoricidal activities).

Indeed macrophages play an important role not only in immunity but also in reorganization of tissues. However, because of their potent activities, macrophage can also do damage to tissues.

Many of these macrophage functions can only be performed by activated macrophages. Macrophage activation can be defined as quantitative alterations in the expression of various gene products that enable the activated macrophage to perform some function that cannot be performed by the resting macrophage.

Macrophage activation is an important function of Th1 cells. When Th1 cells get activated by an APC such as a macrophage, they releases IFN-γ, which is one of two signals required to activate a macrophage. Lipopolysaccharide (LPS) from bacteria or TNF-α produced by macrophages exposed to bacterial products deliver the second signal.

Effector mechanisms employed by macrophages include production of:

- TNF-α, which can induce apoptosis
- Nitric oxide and other reactive nitrogen intermediates
- Reactive oxygen intermediates
- Cationic proteins and hydrolytic enzymes.

Macrophage activation by Th1 cells is very important in protection against many different pathogens For example, Pneumocystis *carinii*, an extracellular pathogen, is controlled in normal individuals by activated macrophages; it is, however, a common cause of death in AIDS patients because they are deficient in Th1 cells. Similarly, *Mycobacterium tuberculosis*, an intracellular pathogen that resides in vesicles, is not efficiently killed by macrophages unless they are activated; hence this infection is a problem in AIDS patients.

Cell-cell Interactions in Cell-mediated Immunity - Activation of NK Cells

Cytokines produced by activated Th1 cells, particularly Il-2 and IFN-γ, also activate NK cells to become lymphokine activated killer cells (LAK cells). LAK cells are able to kill virus infected and tumor cells in a non-MHC-restricted manner.

Indeed, susceptibility of target cells to killing by NK and LAK cells is inversely proportional to the expression of MHC class I molecules.

The effector mechanisms used by NK and LAK cells to kill target cells is similar to those used by CTLs (*e.g.*, perforin and granzymes). NK and LAK cells are also able to kill antibody coated target cells by ADCC.

Chapter

4

Bacteriology

Procaryotic Life

The Bacteria are a group of single-cell microorganisms with procaryotic cellular configuration. The genetic material (DNA) of procaryotic cells exists unbound in the cytoplasm of the cells. There is no nuclear membrane, which is the definitive characteristic of eucaryotic cells such as those that make up, fungi, protista, plants and animals. Until recently, bacteria were the only known type of procaryotic cell, and the discipline of biology related to their study is called bacteriology. In the 1980's, with the outbreak of molecular techniques applied to phylogeny of life, another group of procaryotes was defined and informally named "archaebacteria".

This group of procaryotes has since been renamed Archaea and has been awarded biological Domain status on the level with Bacteria and Eucarya. The current science of bacteriology includes the study of both domains of procaryotic cells, but the name "bacteriology" is not likely to change to reflect the inclusion of archaea in the discipline. Actually, many archaea have been studied as intensively and as long as their bacterial counterparts, except with the notion that they were bacteria.

The Origin of Life

When life arose on Earth about 4 billion years ago, the first types of cells to evolve were procaryotic cells. For approximately 2 billion years, procaryotic-type cells were the only form of life on Earth. The oldest known sedimentary rocks, from Greenland, are about 3.8 billion years old. The oldest known fossils are procaryotic cells, 3.5 billion years in age, found in Western Australia and South Africa. The nature of these fossils, and the chemical composition of the rocks in which they are found, indicates that lithotrophic and fermentative modes of metabolism were the first to evolve in early procaryotes. Photosynthesis developed in bacteria a bit later, at least 3 billion years ago. Anoxygenic photosynthesis (bacterial photosynthesis, which is anaerobic and does not produce O_2) preceded oxygenic photosynthesis (plant-type photosynthesis, which yields O_2).

However, oxygenic photosynthesis also arose in procaryotes, specifically in the cyanobacteria, which existed millions of years before the evolution of green algae and plants. Larger, more complicated eucaryotic cells did not appear until much later, between 1.5 and 2 billion years ago.

The archaea and bacteria differ fundamentally in their structure from eucaryotic cells, which always contain a membrane-enclosed nucleus, multiple chromosomes, and various other membranous organelles such as mitochondria, chloroplasts, the golgi apparatus, vacuoles, etc. Unlike plants and animals, archaea and bacteria are unicellular organisms that do not develop or differentiate into multicellular forms. Some bacteria grow in filaments or masses of cells, but each cell in the colony is identical and capable of independent existence. The cells may be adjacent to one another because they did not separate after cell division or because they remained enclosed in a common sheath or slime secreted by the cells, but typically there is no continuity or communication between the cells.

The Universal Tree of Life

On the basis of small subunit ribosomal RNA (ssrRNA) analysis, the contemporary Tree of Life gives rise to three cellular "Domains": Archaea, Bacteria, and Eucarya. Bacteria (formerly known as eubacteria) and Archaea (formerly called archaebacteria) share the procaryotic type of cellular configuration, but otherwise are not related to one another any more closely than they are to the eucaryotic domain, Eucarya.

Between the two procaryotes, Archaea are apparently more closely related to Eucarya than are the Bacteria. Eucarya consists of all eucaryotic cell-types, including protista, fungi, plants and animals.

Size and Distribution of Bacteria and Archaea

Most procaryotic cells are very small compared to eucaryotic cells. A typical bacterial cell is about 1 micrometer in diameter or width, while most eucaryotic cells are from 10 to 100 micrometers in diameter. Eucaryotic cells have a much greater volume of cytoplasm and a much lower surface: volume ratio than procaryotic cells. A typical procaryotic cell is about the size of a eucaryotic mitochondrion. Since procaryotes are too small to be seen except with the aid of a microscope, it is usually not appreciated that they are the most abundant form of life on the planet, both in terms of biomass and total numbers of species. For example, in the sea, procaryotes make up 90 percent of the total combined weight of all organisms. In a single gram of fertile agricultural soil there may be in excess of 10^9 bacterial cells, outnumbering all eucaryotic cells there by 10,000 : 1. About 3,000 distinct species of bacteria and archaea are recognized, but this number is probably less than one percent of all the species in nature. These unknown procaryotes, far in excess of undiscovered or unstudied plants, are a tremendous reserve of genetic material and genetic information in nature that awaits exploitation. Procaryotes are found in all of the habitats where eucaryotes live, but, as well, in many natural environments considered too extreme or inhospitable for eucaryotic cells. Thus, the outer limits of life on Earth (hottest, coldest, driest, etc.) are usually defined by the existence of procaryotes. Where eucaryotes and procaryotes live together, there may be mutualistic associations between the organisms that allow both to survive or flourish. The organelles of eucaryotes (mitochondria and chloroplasts) are thought to be remnants of Bacteria that invaded, or were captured by, primitive eucaryotes in the evolutionary past. Numerous types of eucaryotic cells that exist today are inhabited by endosymbiotic procaryotes.

From a metabolic standpoint, the procaryotes are extraordinarily diverse, and they exhibit several types of metabolism that are rarely or never seen in eucaryotes. For example, the biological processes of nitrogen fixation (conversion of atmospheric nitrogen gas to ammonia) and methanogenesis (production of methane) are metabolically-unique to procaryotes and have an enormous impact on the nitrogen and carbon cycles in nature. Unique mechanisms for energy production and photosynthesis are also seen among the Archaea and Bacteria.

The lives of plants and animals are dependent upon the activities of bacterial cells. Bacteria and archaea enter into various types of symbiotic relationships with plants and animals that usually benefit both organisms, although a few bacteria are agents of disease. The metabolic activities of procaryotes in soil habitats have an enormous impact on soil fertility that can affect agricultural practices and crop yields. In the global environment, procaryotes are absolutely essential to drive the cycles of elements that make up living systems, i.e., the carbon, oxygen, nitrogen and sulphur cycles. The origins of the plant cell chloroplast and plant-type (oxygenic) photosynthesis are found in procaryotes. Most of the earth's atmospheric oxygen may have been produced by free-living bacterial cells. The bacteria fix nitrogen and a substantial amount of CO_2, as well. Bacteria or bacterial products (including their genes) can be used to increase crop yield or plant resistance to disease, or to cure or prevent plant disease. Bacterial products include antibiotics to fight infectious disease, as well as components for vaccines used to prevent infectious disease. Because of their simplicity and our relative understanding of their biological processes, the bacteria provide convenient laboratory models for study of the molecular biology, genetics, and physiology of all types of cells, including plant and animal cells.

Structure and Function of Procaryotic Cells

Procaryotic cells have three architectural regions: appendages (proteins attached to the cell surface) in the form of flagella and pili; a cell envelope consisting of a capsule, cell wall and plasma membrane; and a cytoplasmic region that contains the cell genome (DNA) and ribosomes and various sorts of inclusions.

Surface Structures-Appendages

Flagella are filamentous protein structures attached to the cell surface that provide swimming movement for most motile procaryotic cells. The flagellar filament is rotated by a motor apparatus in the plasma membrane allowing the cell to swim in fluid environments. Bacterial flagella are powered by proton motive force (chemiosmotic potential) established on the bacterial membrane, rather than ATP hydrolysis which powers eucaryotic flagella and cilia. Procaryotes are known to exhibit a variety of types of tactic behaviour, i.e., the ability to move (swim) in response to environmental stimuli. For example, during chemotaxis a bacterium can sense the quality and quantity of certain chemicals in their environment and swim towards them (if they are useful nutrients) or away from them (if they are harmful substances).

Fimbriae and Pili are interchangeable terms used to designate short, hair-like structures on the surfaces of procaryotic cells. Fimbriae are shorter and stiffer than flagella, and slightly smaller in diameter. Like flagella, they are composed of protein. A specialized type of pilus, the F or sex pilus, in some way stabilizes the transfer of DNA between mating bacteria, but the function of the smaller, more numerous common pili is quite different. Common pili (often called fimbriae) are usually involved in adherence (attachment) of procaryotes to surfaces in nature. In medical situations, they are major determinants of bacterial virulence because they allow pathogens to attach to (colonize) tissues and to resist attack by phagocytic white blood cells.

The Cell Envelope

Most procaryotes have a rigid cell wall. The cell wall is an essential structure that protects the delicate cell protoplast from osmotic lysis. The cell wall of Bacteria consists of a polymer of disaccharides cross-linked by short chains of amino acids (peptides). This molecule is a type of peptidoglycan, which is called murein. In the Gram-positive bacteria (those that retain the purple crystal violet dye when subjected to the Gram-staining procedure) the cell wall is a thick layer of murein. In the Gram-negative bacteria (cells which do not retain the crystal violet dye) the cell wall is relatively thin and is composed of a thin layer of murein surrounded by a membranous structure called the outer membrane.

Murein is a substance unique in nature to bacterial cell walls. Also, the outer membrane of Gram-negative bacteria invariably contains a unique component, lipopolysaccharide (LPS or endotoxin), which is toxic to animals. The cell walls of Archaea may be composed of protein, polysaccharides, or peptidgolycan-like molecules, but never do they contain murein. This feature distinguishes the Bacteria from the Archaea.

Although procaryotes lack any intracellular organelles for respiration or photosynthesis, many species possess the physiologic ability to conduct these processes, usually as a function of their plasma membrane. For example, the electron transport system that couples aerobic respiration and ATP synthesis is found in the plasma membrane. The photosynthetic chromophores that harvest light energy for conversion into chemical energy are located in the membrane. Hence, the plasma membrane is the site of oxidative phosphorylation and photophosphorylation in procaryotes, analogous to the functions of mitochondria and chloroplasts in eucaryotic cells. The procaryotic plasma membrane is also a permeability barrier, and it contains a variety of different transport systems that selectively mediate the passage of substances into and out of the cell.

The membranes of Bacteria are structurally similar to the cell membranes of eucaryotes, except that bacterial membranes consist of saturated or monounsaturated fatty acids (rarely polyunsaturated fatty acids) and do not normally contain sterols. The membranes of Archaea form phospholipid bilayers functionally equivalent to bacterial membranes, but archaeal lipids are saturated, branched, repeating isoprenoid subunits that attach to glycerol via an ether linkage, as opposed to the ester linkage found in glycerides of eucaryotic and bacterial membrane lipids. The structure of archaeal membranes is thought to be an adaptation to their existence in extreme environments.

Most bacteria contain some sort of a polysaccharide layer outside of the cell wall or outer membrane. In a general sense, this layer is called a capsule or glycocalyx. Bacteria and archaea may also have an additional proteinaceous coat called an S-layer. Capsules, slime layers, glycocalyx and s-layer are known to mediate attachment of bacterial cells to particular surfaces. Capsules also protect bacteria from engulfment by predatory protozoa or white blood cells (phagocytes) and from attack by antimicrobial agents of plant or animal origin. Capsules in certain soil bacteria protect them from perennial effects of drying or desiccation.

Importance of Surface Components

All of the various surface components of a procaryotic cell are important in its ecology since they mediate the contact of the cell with its environment.

The only "sense" that a procaryote has results from its immediate contact with its environment. It must use its surface components to assess the environment and respond in a way that supports its own existence and survival in that environment. The surface properties of a procaryote are determined by the exact molecular composition of its plasma membrane cell wall, including LPS, and the function of surface structures such as flagella, fimbriae and capsules. Some important ways that procaryotes use their surface components are (1) as permeability barriers that allow selective passage of nutrients and exclusion of harmful substances; (2) as "adhesins" used to attach or adhere to specific surfaces or tissues; (3) for protection against engulfment by phagocytic white blood cells or predatory protozoa: (4) as enzymes to mediate specific reactions on the cell surface important in the survival of the procaryote; (5) as "sensing proteins" that can respond to temperature, osmolarity, salinity, light, oxygen, nutrients, etc. resulting in a signal to the genome of the cell that will cause a biological response to a changing environment.

Cytoplasmic Constituents

The cytoplasmic constituents of bacteria invariably include the procaryotic chromosome and ribosomes. The chromosome is typically one large circular molecule of DNA, more or less free in the cytoplasm, although intermittently associated with membranes. Procaryotes sometimes possess smaller extrachromosomal pieces of DNA called plasmids. The total DNA content of a cell is referred to as the cell genome. During cell growth and division, the procaryotic chromosome is replicated in the usual semi-conservative fashion before for distribution to progeny cells. However, the eucaryotic processes of meiosis and mitosis are absent in procaryotes. Replication and segregation of procaryotic DNA is coordinated by the plasma membrane.

The distinct granular appearance of procaryotic cytoplasm is due to the presence and distribution of ribosomes The ribosomes of procaryotes are smaller than cytoplasmic ribosomes of eucaryotes. Procaryotic ribosomes are 70S in size, being composed of 30S and 50S subunits.

The 80S ribosomes of eucaryotes are made up of 40S and 60S subunits. Ribosomes are involved in the process of translation (protein synthesis), but some details of their activities differ in eucaryotes, Bacteria and Archaea. Protein synthesis using bacterial 70S ribosomes occurs in eucaryotic mitochondria and chloroplasts, and this is taken as a major line of evidence that these organelles are descended from bacteria.

Often contained in the cytoplasm of procaryotic cells is one or another of some type of inclusion granule. Inclusions are distinct granules that may occupy a substantial part of the cytoplasm. Inclusion granules are usually reserve materials of some sort. For example, carbon and energy reserves may be stored as glycogen (a polymer of glucose) or as polybetahydroxybutyric acid (a type of fat) granules. Polyphosphate inclusions are reserves of PO_4 and possibly energy; elemental sulphur (sulphur globules) are stored by some phototrophic and some lithotrophic procaryotes as reserves of energy or electrons. Some inclusion bodies are actually membranous vesicles or intrusions into the cytoplasm which contain photosynthetic pigments or specialized enzyme complexes.

Taxonomy and Classification of Procaryotes

Haeckel (1866) was the first to create a natural Kingdom for the microorganisms, which had been discovered nearly two centuries before by van Leeuwenhoek. He placed all unicellular (microscopic) organisms in a new kingdom, "Protista", separated from plants (Plantae) and animals (Animalia), which were multicellular (macroscopic) organisms. The development of the electron microscope in the 1950's revealed a fundamental dichotomy among Haeckel's "Protista": some cells contained a membrane-enclosed nucleus, and some cells lacked this intracellular structure.

The latter were temporarily shifted to a fourth kingdom, Monera (or Moneres), the procaryotes (also called Procaryotae). Protista remained as a kingdom of unicellular eucaryotic microorganisms. Whittaker refined the system into five kingdoms in 1967, by identifying the Fungi as a separate multicellular eucaryotic kingdom of organisms, distinguished by their absorptive mode of heterotrophic nutrition.

In the 1980's, Woese began phylogenetic analysis of all forms of cellular life based on comparative sequencing of the small subunit ribosomal RNA (ssrRNA) that is contained in all organisms. A new dichotomy was revealed, this time among the procaryotes: there existed two types of procaryotes, as fundamentally unrelated to one another as they are to eucaryotes. Whittaker's Plant, Animal and Fungal Kingdoms (all of the multicellular eucaryotes) are at the end of a very small branch of the tree of life, and all other branches lead to microorganisms, either procaryotes (Bacteria and Archaea), or protists (unicellular algae and protozoa), thus establishing clearly that microbial life is the predominant form of life on the planet. Sequence analysis of macromolecules such as the small subunit ribosomal RNA found in all cells has allowed bacteriologists to classify bacteria into a typical hierarchal scheme based on genetic relatedness. The current edition (2001) of Bergey's Manual of Systematic Bacteriology has established 24 phyla of bacteria, systematically ordered into class, order, family, genus and species.

For example, *E. coli* is in the Domain Bacteria, Phylum *Proteobacteria*, Class *Gamma Proteobacteria*, Order *Enterobacteriales*, Family *Enterobacteriaceae*, Genus *Escherichia*, Species *E. coli*. You can download Bergey's 400-page taxonomic outline of the procaryotes at Bergey's Manual of Systematic Bacteriology 2nd ed (2001), or you can back in to a taxonomic outline of bacteria in Wikipedia by looking up the scientific name of any well-known bacterium and viewing the right-hand frame, Scientific classification. Although the definitive difference between Woese's Archaea and Bacteria is based on fundamental differences in the nucleotide base sequence in the 16S ribosomal RNA, there are many biochemical and phenotypic differences between the two groups of procaryotes. The phylogenetic tree indicates that Archaea are more closely related to Eucarya than are Bacteria.

This relatedness seems most evident in the similarities between transcription and translation in the Archaea and the Eucarya. However, it is also evident that the Bacteria have evolved into chloroplasts and mitochondria, so that these eucaryotic organelles derive their lineage from this group of procaryotes. Perhaps the biological success of eucaryotic cells springs from the evolutionary merger of the two procaryotic life forms.

Identification of Bacteria

Classic Methods

The criteria used for microscopic identification of procaryotes include cell shape and grouping, Gram-stain reaction, and motility. Bacterial cells almost invariably take one of three forms: rod (bacillus), sphere (coccus), or spiral (spirilla and spirochetes). Rods that are curved are called vibrios.

Fixed bacterial cells stain either Gram-positive (purple) or Gram-negative (pink); motility is easily determined by observing living specimens. Bacilli may occur singly or form chains of cells; cocci may form chains (streptococci) or grape-like clusters (staphylococci); spiral shape cells are almost always motile; cocci are almost never motile. This nomenclature ignores the actinomycetes, a prominent group of branched bacteria which occur in the soil. But they are easily recognized by their colonies and their microscopic appearance.

Such easily-made microscopic observations, combined with knowing the natural environment of the organism, are important aids to identify the group, if not the exact genus, of a bacterium - providing, of course, that one has an effective key. Such a key is Bergey's Manual of Determinative Bacteriology 9th ed, the "field guide" to identification of the bacteria. Bergey's Manual describes affiliated groups of Bacteria and Archaea based on a few easily observed microscopic and physiologic characteristics. Further identification requires biochemical tests which will distinguish genera among families and species among genera. Strains within a single species are usually distinguished by genetic or immunological criteria.

Molecular Techniques

The sciences of genomics and bioinformatics have led to a radical reclassification of procaryotes based on comparative analysis of organismal DNA. Genomics involves the study of all of the nucleotide sequences, including structural genes, regulatory sequences, and noncoding DNA segments, in the chromosomes of an organism.

To date over 200 bacterial genomes have been sequenced. We have seen how highly conserved genetic sequences, such as those that encode for the small subunit ribosomal RNAs (16S rRNA) of an organism, can be analyzed to specifically relate two organisms. So can the identification of certain genes provide information about specific properties of an organism, and analysis of specific nucleotide sequences may be used to indicate identity and degrees of genetic relatedness among organisms.

The newest editions of Bergey's Manual are adapted to the new phylogenetic classification. This has resulted in the formation of several new taxa of bacteria and archaea at every hierarchical level. Occasionally, organisms thought to be more or less distantly related become unified; but more likely, organisms thought to be closely-related due to similar phenotypic properties are found to be genetically distinct and warrant separation into a new taxa.

Metagenomics. Sequencing of 16S rRNA genes obtained from environmental samples produces a broad profile of microbial diversity and reveals that the vast majority of microbes present have been missed by reliance on cultivation-based methods. This observation has given rise to the field of metagenomics. Metagenomics (also called environmental genomics) is the application of modern genomics techniques to the study of communities of microorganisms directly in their natural environments, bypassing the need for isolation and lab cultivation of individual species. Metagenomics provides a means to identify and quantify microbes from environmental samples based on the presence of distinctive genes. This enables studies of organisms that are not easily cultured in the laboratory, as well as studies of organisms in their natural environment. "Shotgun" metagenomics is capable of sequencing nearly complete microbial genomes directly from the environment. Because the collection of DNA from an environment is largely uncontrolled, the most abundant organisms in a sample are most highly represented in the resulting sequence data. To achieve the high coverage needed to fully resolve the genomes of underrepresented community members, large samples, often prohibitively so, may be needed. However, the random nature of shotgun sequencing ensures that many of these organisms will be represented by at least some small sequence segments. Due to the limitations of microbial isolation methods, the majority of these organisms would go unnoticed using traditional culturing techniques.

Shotgun sequencing and screens of clone libraries reveal genes present in environmental samples. This provides information both on which organisms are present and what metabolic processes are possible in the community. This can be helpful in understanding the ecology of a community, particularly if multiple samples are compared to one other.

Bacterial Reproduction and Genetics

Most bacteria reproduce by a relatively simple asexual process called binary fission: each cell increases in size and divides into two cells. During this process there is an orderly increase in cellular structures and components, replication and segregation of the bacterial DNA, followed by formation of a septum or cross wall which divides the cell into two. The process is evidently coordinated by activities associated with the cell membrane. The DNA molecule is believed to be attached to a point on the membrane where it is replicated. The two DNA molecules remain attached at points side-by-side on the membrane while new membrane material is synthesized between the two points. This draws the DNA molecules in opposite directions while new cell wall and membrane are laid down as a septum between the two chromosomal compartments. When septum formation is complete the cell splits into two progeny cells. The time interval required for a bacterial cell to divide or for a population of cells to double is called the generation time. Generation times for bacterial species growing in nature may be as short as 15 minutes or as long as several days.

Genetic Exchange in Bacteria

Although procaryotes do not undergo sexual reproduction, they are not without the ability to exchange genes and undergo genetic recombination. Bacteria are known to exchange genes in nature by three fundamental processes: conjugation, transduction and transformation. Conjugation requires cell-to-cell contact for DNA to be transferred from a donor to a recipient. During transduction, a virus transfers the genes between mating bacteria. In transformation, DNA is acquired directly from the environment, having been released from another cell. Genetic recombination can follow the transfer of

DNA from one cell to another leading to the emergence of a new genotype (recombinant). It is common for DNA to be transferred as plasmids between mating bacteria. Since bacteria usually develop their genes for drug resistance on plasmids (called resistance transfer factors, or RTFs), they are able to spread drug resistance to other strains and species during genetic exchange processes.

The genetic engineering of bacterial cells in the research or biotechnology laboratory is often based on the use of plasmids as vectors. The genetic systems of the Archaea are poorly characterized at this point, although the entire genome of *Methanosarcina* has been sequenced which opens up the possibilities for genetic analysis of the group.

Evolution of Bacteria and Archaea

For most procaryotes, mutation is a major source of variability that allows the species to adapt to new conditions. The mutation rate for most procaryotic genes is in the neighborhood of 10^{-8}. This means that if a bacterial population doubles from 10^8 cells to 2×10^8 cells, there is likely to be a mutant present for any given gene. Since procaryotes grow to reach population densities far in excess of 10^9 cells, such a mutant could develop from a single generation during 15 minutes of growth. The evolution of procaryotes, driven by such Darwinian principles of evolution (mutation and selection) is called vertical evolution.

However, as a result of the processes of genetic exchange described above, the bacteria and archaea can also undergo a process of horizontal evolution, also called horizontal gene transfer (HGT). In this case, genes are transferred laterally from one organism to another, including between members of different Kingdoms, which allows the recipient to experiment with a new genetic trait. Horizontal gene transfer is becoming realized to be a significant force in driving cellular evolution.

The combined effects of fast growth rates, high concentrations of cells, genetic processes of mutation and selection, and the ability to exchange genes, account for the extraordinary rates of adaptation and evolution that can be observed in the procaryotes.

Ecology of Bacteria and Archaea

Bacteria and Archaea are present in all environments that support life. They may be free-living, or living in associations with "higher forms" of life (plants and animals), and they are found in environments that support no other form of life. Procaryotes have the usual nutritional requirements for growth of cells, but many of the ways that they utilize and transform their nutrients are unique. This bears directly on their habitat and their ecology.

Nutritional Types of Organisms

In terms of carbon utilization a cell may be heterotrophic or autotrophic. Heterotrophs obtain their carbon and energy for growth from organic compounds in nature. Autotrophs use $C0_2$ as a sole source of carbon for growth and obtain their energy from light (e.g. photoautotrophs) or from the oxidation of inorganic compounds (e.g. lithoautotrophs).

Most heterotrophic bacteria are saprophytes, meaning that they obtain their nourishment from dead organic matter. In the soil, saprophytic bacteria and fungi are responsible for biodegradation of organic material. Ultimately, organic molecules, no matter how complex, can be degraded to CO_2 (plus H_2 and H_2O). Probably no naturally-occurring organic substance cannot be degraded by the combined activities of the bacteria and fungi. Hence, most organic matter in nature is converted by heterotrophs to CO_2, only to be converted back into organic material by autotrophs that die and nourish heterotrophs to complete the carbon cycle.

Lithotrophic procaryotes have a type of energy-producing metabolism which is unique. Lithotrophs (also called lithoautotrophs or chemoautotrophs) use inorganic compounds as sources of energy, i.e., they oxidize compounds such as H_2 or H_2S or NH_3 to obtain electrons to feed in to an electron transport system and to produce ATP.

Lithotrophs are found in soil and aquatic environments wherever their energy source is present. Most lithotrophs are autotrophs so they can grow in the absence of any organic material. Lithotrophic species are found among the Bacteria and the Archaea. Sulphur-oxidizing lithotrophs convert H_2S to S^o and S^o to SO_4. Nitrifying bacteria convert NH_3 to NO_2 and NO_2 to NO_3; methanogenic archaea strip electrons off of H_2 as a source of energy and add them to CO_2 to form CH_4 (methane). Lithotrophs have an obvious impact on the sulphur, nitrogen and carbon cycles in the biosphere.

Photosynthetic bacteria convert light energy into chemical energy for growth. Most phototrophic bacteria are autotrophs so their role in the carbon cycle is analogous to that of plants. The planktonic cyanobacteria are the "grass of the sea" and their form of oxygenic photosynthesis generates a substantial amount of O_2 in the biosphere. However, among the photosynthetic bacteria are types of photosynthetic metabolism not seen in eucaryotes, including photoheterotrophy (using light as an energy source while assimilating organic compounds as a source of carbon), anoxygenic photosynthesis, and unique mechanisms of CO_2 fixation (autotrophy).

Photosynthesis has not been found to occur among the Archaea, but one archaeal species employs a light-driven non photosynthetic means of energy generation based on the use of a chromophore called bacteriorhodopsin.

Adaptations to Environmental Conditions

Most procaryotes, whether they have been cultured and studied in the laboratory, or observed growing in their natural habitats, seem to be highly adapted to their specific environment by means of their macromolecular structure and/or their physiologic (metabolic) capabilities. The nutritional quality of the environment determines whether a particular organism will be present, but so do various physical parameters such as the availability of light and O_2, as well as the pH, temperature and salinity of the environment. As examples, the range of procaryotic responses to oxygen and temperature are discussed below.

Procaryotes vary widely in their response to O_2 (molecular oxygen). Organisms that require O_2 for growth are called obligate aerobes; those which are inhibited or killed by O_2, and which grow only in its absence, are called obligate anaerobes; organisms which grow either in the presence or absence of O_2 are called facultative anaerobes. Whether or not a particular organism can exist in the presence of O_2 depends upon the distribution of certain enzymes such as superoxide dismutase and catalase that are required to detoxify lethal oxygen radicals that are always generated by living systems in the presence of O_2

Procaryotes also vary widely in their response to temperature. Those that live at very cold temperatures (0 degrees or lower) are called psychrophiles; those which flourish at room temperature (25 degrees) or at the temperature of warm-blooded animals (37 degrees) are called mesophiles; those that live at high temperatures (greater than 45 degrees) are thermophiles. The only limit that seems to be placed on growth of certain procaryotes in nature relative to temperature is whether liquid water exists. Hence, growing procaryotic cells can be found in supercooled environments (ice does not form) as low as -20 degrees and superheated environments (steam does not form) as high as 120 degrees. Archaea have been detected around thermal vents on the ocean floor where the temperature is as high as 320 degrees!

Symbiosis

The biomass of procaryotic cells in the biosphere, their metabolic diversity, and their persistence in all habitats that support life, ensures that these microbe will play a crucial role in the cycles of elements and the functioning of the world ecosystem. However, the procaryotes affect the world ecology in another significant way through their inevitable interactions with insects, plants and animals. Some bacteria are required to associate with insects, animals or plants for the latter to survive. For example, the sex of offspring of certain insects is determined by endosymbiotic bacteria. Ruminant animals (cows, sheep, etc.), whose diet is mainly cellulose (plant material), must have cellulose-digesting bacteria in their intestine to convert the cellulose to a form of carbon that the animal can assimilate. Leguminous plants grow poorly in nitrogen-deprived soils unless they are colonized by nitrogen-fixing bacteria which can supply them with a biologically-useful form of nitrogen.

Bacterial Pathogenicity

Some bacteria are parasites of plants or animals, meaning that they grow at the expense of their eucaryotic host and may damage, harm, or even kill it in the process. Such bacteria that cause disease in plants or animals are pathogens. Human diseases caused by bacterial pathogens include tuberculosis, whooping cough, diphtheria, tetanus, gonorrhea, syphilis, pneumonia, cholera and typhoid fever, to name a few. The bacteria that cause these diseases have special structural or biochemical properties that determine their virulence or pathogenicity. These include: (1) ability to colonize and invade their host; (2) ability to resist or withstand the antibacterial defenses of the host; (3) ability to produce various toxic substances that damage the host. Plant diseases, likewise, may be caused by bacterial pathogens. More than 200 species of bacteria are associated with plant diseases, but a very small handful of genera are involved.

Chapter

5

Applications of Bacteria in Industry and Biotechnology

Exploitation of Bacteria by Humans

Bacteria are used in industry in a number of ways that generally exploit their natural metabolic capabilities. They are used in manufacture of foods and production of antibiotics, probiotics, drugs, vaccines, starter cultures, insecticides, enzymes, fuels and solvents. In addition, with genetic engineering technology, bacteria can be programmed to make various substances used in food science, agriculture and medicine. The genetic systems of bacteria are the foundation of the biotechnology industry discussed below.

In the foods industry, lactic acid bacteria such as *Lactobacillus, Lactococcus* and *Streptococcus* are used in the manufacture of dairy products such as cheeses, including cottage cheese and cream cheese, cultured butter, sour cream, buttermilk, yogurt and kefir. Lactic acid bacteria and acetic acid bacteria are used in pickling processes such as olives, cucumber pickles and sauerkraut. Bacterial fermentations are used in processing of teas, coffee, cocoa, soy sauce, sausages and an amazing variety of foods in our everyday lives. In the pharmaceutical industry, bacteria are used to produce antibiotics, vaccines, and medically-useful enzymes. Most antibiotics are made by bacteria that live in soil. Actinomycetes such as *Streptomyces* produce tetracyclines, erythromycin, streptomycin, rifamycin and ivermectin. *Bacillus* and

Paenibacillus species produce bacitracin and polymyxin. Bacterial products are used in the manufacture of vaccines for immunization against infectious disease. Vaccines against diphtheria, whooping cough, tetanus, typhoid fever and cholera are made from components of the bacteria that cause the respective diseases. It is significant to note here that the use of antibiotics against infectious disease and the widespread practice of vaccination (immunization) against infectious disease are two twentieth-century developments that have drastically increased the quality of life and the average life expectancy of individuals in developed countries.

Biotechnology

The biotechnology industry uses bacterial cells for the production of biological substances that are useful to human existence, including fuels, foods, medicines, hormones, enzymes, proteins, and nucleic acids. The possibilities of biotechnology are endless considering the gene reservoirs and genetic capabilities within the bacteria. Pasteur said it best, "Never underestimate the power of the microbe." Biotechnology has produced human hormones such as insulin, enzymes such as streptokinase, and human proteins such as interferon and tumor necrosis factor. These products are used for the treatment of a various medical conditions and diseases including diabetes, heart attack, tuberculosis, AIDS and SLE. Botulinum toxin and BT insecticide are bacterial products used in medicine and pest control, respectively. One biotechnological application of bacteria involves the genetic construction of super strains of organisms to perform particular metabolic tasks in the environment. For example, bacteria which have been engineered genetically to degrade petroleum products are used in cleanup of oil spills and other bioremediation efforts. Another area of biotechnology involves improvement of the qualities of plants through genetic engineering. Genes can be introduced into plants by a bacterium *Agrobacterium tumefaciens*. Using *A. tumefaciens*, plants have been genetically engineered so that they are resistant to certain pests, herbicides, and diseases.

Finally, it should not be overlooked that industrial, pharmaceutical and food microbiology are applications of biotechnology. Archaea and bacteria are involved in production of biofuels. Bacteria are the main producers of clinically useful antibiotics; they are a source of vaccines against once dreaded diseases; they are probiotics that enhance our health; and they are primary participants in the fermentations of dairy products and many other foods.

General Characteristics of Bacteria

Bacteria are prokaryotes, i.e. they do not have their DNA enclosed in a nucleus (Bacteria, 2005). They are among the earliest life forms that appeared on Earth billions of years ago, and helped change the environment, creating oxygen which enabled higher forms to evolve. The Universal Tree of Life derived from sequencing ssrRNA gives three major domains of living organisms: Eucarya, Archaea and Bacteria (Todar, 2005).

Although there are thousands of different bacteria, they come in three basic forms: rod shaped, called bacilli; round, ball-shaped forms called cocci); and some are spiral in shape. Bacterial cells can exist as individual cells, or may group together in chains (rods and cocci) or cocci can aggregate in clusters. They have a cell envelope consisting of a capsule, the cell wall, and a plasma membrane, and a cytoplasmic region which contains the cell genome (DNA), ribosomes, and various cell inclusions. (Todar, 2005).

Most bacteria have a rigid cell wall which protects the cell protoplast from osmotic lysis, and consists of a polymer of disaccharides cross-linked by short amino acid chains (peptides) forming a peptidoglycans called mucin. Gram-positive bacteria (those that retain the purple dye) have a cell wall with a thick layer of murein. Gram-negative bacteria, which exclude the dye, have a relatively thin cell wall composed of murein surrounded by a membranous structure called the outer membrane. Murein is unique to bacterial cell walls.

Bacteria are a large group of single-celled, prokaryote microorganisms. Typically a few micrometres in length, bacteria have a wide range of shapes, ranging from spheres to rods and spirals. Bacteria are ubiquitous in every habitat on Earth, growing in soil, acidic hot springs, radioactive waste, water, and deep in the Earth's crust, as well as in organic matter and the live bodies of plants and animals.

There are typically 40 million bacterial cells in a gram of soil and a million bacterial cells in a millilitre of fresh water; in all, there are approximately five nonillion (5×10^{30}) bacteria on Earth, forming much of the world's biomass. Bacteria are vital in recycling nutrients, with many steps in nutrient cycles depending on these organisms, such as the fixation of nitrogen from the atmosphere and putrefaction. However, most bacteria have not been characterised, and only about half of the phyla of bacteria have species that can be grown in the laboratory. The study of bacteria is known as bacteriology, a branch of microbiology.

There are approximately ten times as many bacterial cells in the human flora as there are human cells in the body, with large numbers of bacteria on the skin and as gut flora. The vast majority of the bacteria in the body are rendered harmless by the protective effects of the immune system, and a few are beneficial. However, a few species of bacteria are pathogenic and cause infectious diseases, including cholera, syphilis, anthrax, leprosy and bubonic plague.

The most common fatal bacterial diseases are respiratory infections, with tuberculosis alone killing about 2 million people a year, mostly in sub-Saharan Africa. In developed countries, antibiotics are used to treat bacterial infections and in agriculture, so antibiotic resistance is becoming common. In industry, bacteria are important in sewage treatment, the production of cheese and yogurt through fermentation, as well as in biotechnology, and the manufacture of antibiotics and other chemicals.

Once regarded as plants constituting the Class Schizomycetes, bacteria are now classified as prokaryotes. Unlike cells of animals and other eukaryotes, bacterial cells do not contain a nucleus and rarely harbour membrane-bound organelles. Although the term *bacteria* traditionally included all prokaryotes, the scientific classification changed after the discovery in the 1990s that prokaryotes consist of two very different groups of organisms that evolved independently from an ancient common ancestor. These evolutionary domains are called Bacteria and Archaea.

Bacteria display a wide diversity of shapes and sizes, called *morphologies*. Bacterial cells are about one tenth the size of eukaryotic cells and are typically 0.5–5.0 micrometres in length. However, a few species–for example *Thiomargarita namibiensis* and *Epulopiscium fishelsoni*–are up to half a millimetre long and are visible to the unaided eye. Among the smallest bacteria are members of the genus *Mycoplasma*, which measure only 0.3 micrometres, as small as the largest viruses. Some bacteria may be even smaller, but these ultramicrobacteria are not well-studied.

Most bacterial species are either spherical, called cocci or rod-shaped, called bacilli (*sing.* bacillus, from Latin *baculus*, stick). Elongation is associated with swimming. Some rod-shaped bacteria, called vibrio, are slightly curved or comma-shaped; others, can be spiral-shaped, called spirilla, or tightly coiled, called spirochaetes. A small number of species even have tetrahedral or cuboidal shapes.

More recently, bacteria were discovered deep under the Earth's crust that grow as long rods with a star-shaped cross-section. The large surface area to volume ratio of this morphology may give these bacteria an advantage in nutrient-poor environments. This wide variety of shapes is determined by the bacterial cell wall and cytoskeleton, and is important because it can influence the ability of bacteria to acquire nutrients, attach to surfaces, swim through liquids and escape predators.

Many bacterial species exist simply as single cells, others associate in characteristic patterns: *Neisseria* form diploids (pairs), *Streptococcus* form chains, and *Staphylococcus* group together in "bunch of grapes" clusters. Bacteria can also be elongated to form filaments, for example the Actinobacteria. Filamentous bacteria are often surrounded by a sheath that contains many individual cells. Certain types, such as species of the genus *Nocardia*, even form complex, branched filaments, similar in appearance to fungal mycelia. Bacteria often attach to surfaces and form dense aggregations called biofilms or bacterial mats. These films can range from a few micrometers in thickness to up to half a meter in depth, and may contain multiple species of bacteria, protists and archaea. Bacteria living in biofilms display a complex arrangement of cells and extracellular components, forming secondary structures such as microcolonies, through which there are networks of channels to enable better diffusion of nutrients.

In natural environments, such as soil or the surfaces of plants, the majority of bacteria are bound to surfaces in biofilms. Biofilms are also important in medicine, as these structures are often present during chronic bacterial infections or in infections of implanted medical devices, and bacteria protected within biofilms are much harder to kill than individual isolated bacteria. Even more complex morphological changes are sometimes possible. For example, when starved of amino acids, Myxobacteria detect surrounding cells in a process known as quorum sensing, migrate towards each other, and aggregate to form fruiting bodies up to 500 micrometres long and containing approximately 100,000 bacterial cells. In these fruiting bodies, the bacteria perform separate tasks; this type of cooperation is a simple type of multicellular organisation. For example, about one in 10 cells migrate to the top of these fruiting bodies and differentiate into a specialised dormant state called myxospores, which are more resistant to drying and other adverse environmental conditions than are ordinary cells.

Cellular Structure

Intracellular Structures: The bacterial cell is surrounded by a lipid membrane, or cell membrane, which encloses the contents of the cell and acts as a barrier to hold nutrients, proteins and other essential components of the cytoplasm within the cell. As they are prokaryotes, bacteria do not tend to have membrane-bound organelles in their cytoplasm and thus contain few large intracellular structures. They consequently lack a nucleus, mitochondria, chloroplasts and the other organelles present in eukaryotic cells, such as the Golgi apparatus and endoplasmic reticulum. Bacteria were once seen as simple bags of cytoplasm, but elements such as prokaryotic cytoskeleton, and the localization of proteins to specific locations within the cytoplasm have been found to show levels of complexity. These subcellular compartments have been called "bacterial hyperstructures".

Micro-compartments such as carboxysome provides a further level of organization, which are compartments within bacteria that are surrounded by polyhedral protein shells, rather than by lipid membranes. These "polyhedral organelles" localize and compartmentalize bacterial metabolism, a function performed by the membrane-bound organelles in eukaryotes. Many important biochemical reactions, such as energy generation, occur by concentration gradients across membranes, a potential difference also found in a battery. The general lack of internal membranes in bacteria means reactions such as electron transport occur across the cell membrane between the cytoplasm and the periplasmic space. However, in many photosynthetic bacteria the plasma membrane is highly folded and fills most of the cell with layers of light-gathering membrane. These light-gathering complexes may even form lipid-enclosed structures called chlorosomes in green sulphur bacteria. Other proteins import nutrients across the cell membrane, or to expel undesired molecules from the cytoplasm.

Bacteria do not have a membrane-bound nucleus, and their genetic material is typically a single circular chromosome located in the cytoplasm in an irregularly shaped body called the nucleoid. The nucleoid contains the chromosome with associated proteins and RNA. The order Planctomycetes are an exception to the general absence of internal membranes in bacteria, because they have a membrane around their nucleoid and contain other membrane-bound cellular structures. Like all living organisms, bacteria contain ribosomes for the production of proteins, but the structure of the bacterial ribosome is different from those of eukaryotes and Archaea. Some bacteria produce intracellular nutrient storage granules, such as glycogen, polyphosphate, sulphur or polyhydroxyalkanoates. These granules enable bacteria to store compounds for later use. Certain bacterial species, such as the photosynthetic Cyanobacteria, produce internal gas vesicles, which they use to regulate their buoyancy – allowing them to move up or down into water layers with different light intensities and nutrient levels.

Extracellular Structures: Around the outside of the cell membrane is the bacterial cell wall. Bacterial cell walls are made of peptidoglycan (called murein in older sources), which is made from polysaccharide chains cross-linked by unusual peptides containing D-amino acids. Bacterial cell walls are different from the cell walls of plants and fungi, which are made of cellulose and chitin, respectively. The cell wall of bacteria is also distinct from that of Archaea, which do not contain peptidoglycan. The cell wall is essential to the survival of many bacteria, and the antibiotic penicillin is able to kill bacteria by inhibiting a step in the synthesis of peptidoglycan.

There are broadly speaking two different types of cell wall in bacteria, called Gram-positive and Gram-negative. The names originate from the reaction of cells to the Gram stain, a test long-employed for the classification of bacterial species.

Gram-positive bacteria possess a thick cell wall containing many layers of peptidoglycan and teichoic acids. In contrast, Gram-negative bacteria have a relatively thin cell wall consisting of a few layers of peptidoglycan surrounded by a second lipid membrane containing lipopolysaccharides and lipoproteins. Most bacteria have the Gram-negative cell wall, and only the Firmicutes and Actinobacteria (previously known as the low G+C and high G+C Gram-positive bacteria, respectively) have the alternative Gram-positive arrangement. These differences in structure can produce differences in antibiotic susceptibility; for instance, vancomycin can kill only Gram-positive bacteria and is ineffective against Gram-negative pathogens, such as *Haemophilus influenzae* or *Pseudomonas aeruginosa*.

In many bacteria an S-layer of rigidly arrayed protein molecules covers the outside of the cell. This layer provides chemical and physical protection for the cell surface and can act as a macromolecular diffusion barrier. S-layers have diverse but mostly poorly understood functions, but are known to act as virulence factors in *Campylobacter* and contain surface enzymes in *Bacillus stearothermophilus*. Flagella are rigid protein structures, about 20 nanometres in diameter and up to 20 micrometres in length, that are used for motility. Flagella are driven by the energy released by the transfer of ions down an electrochemical gradient across the cell membrane. Fimbriae are fine filaments of protein, just 2–10 nanometres in diameter and up to several micrometers in length. They are distributed over the surface of the cell, and resemble fine hairs when seen under the electron microscope. Fimbriae are believed to be involved in attachment to solid surfaces or to other cells and are essential for the virulence of some bacterial pathogens. Pili (*sing.* pilus) are cellular appendages, slightly larger than fimbriae, that can transfer genetic material between bacterial cells in a process called conjugation.

Capsules or slime layers are produced by many bacteria to surround their cells, and vary in structural complexity: ranging from a disorganised slime layer of extra-cellular polymer, to a highly structured capsule or glycocalyx. These structures can protect cells from engulfment by eukaryotic cells, such as macrophages. They can also act as antigens and be involved in cell recognition, as well as aiding attachment to surfaces and the formation of biofilms. The assembly of these extracellular structures is dependent on bacterial secretion systems. These transfer proteins from the cytoplasm into the periplasm or into the environment around the cell. Many types of secretion systems are known and these structures are often essential for the virulence of pathogens, so are intensively studied.

Endospores

Certain genera of Gram-positive bacteria, such as *Bacillus*, *Clostridium*, *Sporohalobacter*, *Anaerobacter* and *Heliobacterium*, can form highly resistant, dormant structures called endospores. In almost all cases, one endospore is formed and this is not a reproductive process, although *Anaerobacter* can make up to seven endospores in a single cell. Endospores have a central core of cytoplasm containing DNA and ribosomes surrounded by a cortex layer and protected by an impermeable and rigid coat.

Endospores show no detectable metabolism and can survive extreme physical and chemical stresses, such as high levels of UV light, gamma radiation, detergents, disinfectants, heat, freezing, pressure and desiccation. In this dormant state, these organisms may remain viable for millions of years, and endospores even allow bacteria to survive exposure to the vacuum and radiation in space. Endospore-forming bacteria can also cause disease: for example, anthrax can be contracted by the inhalation of *Bacillus anthracis* endospores, and contamination of deep puncture wounds with *Clostridium tetani* endospores causes tetanus.

Metabolism

Bacteria exhibit an extremely wide variety of metabolic types. The distribution of metabolic traits within a group of bacteria has traditionally been used to define their taxonomy, but these traits often do not correspond with modern genetic classifications. Bacterial metabolism is classified into nutritional groups on the basis of three major criteria: the kind of energy used for growth, the source of carbon, and the electron donors used for growth. An additional criterion of respiratory microorganisms are the electron acceptors used for aerobic or anaerobic respiration.

Carbon metabolism in bacteria is either heterotrophic, where organic carbon compounds are used as carbon sources, or autotrophic, meaning that cellular carbon is obtained by fixing carbon dioxide. Heterotrophic bacteria include parasitic types. Typical autotrophic bacteria are phototrophic cyanobacteria, green sulphur-bacteria and some purple bacteria, but also many chemolithotrophic species, such as nitrifying or sulphur-oxidising bacteria. Energy metabolism of bacteria is either based on phototrophy, the use of light through photosynthesis, or on chemotrophy, the use of chemical substances for energy, which are mostly oxidised at the expense of oxygen or alternative electron acceptors (aerobic/anaerobic respiration).

Finally, bacteria are further divided into lithotrophs that use inorganic electron donors and organotrophs that use organic compounds as electron donors. Chemotrophic organisms use the respective electron donors for energy conservation (by aerobic/anaerobic respiration or fermentation) and biosynthetic reactions (e.g. carbon dioxide fixation), whereas phototrophic organisms use them only for biosynthetic purposes.

Respiratory organisms use chemical compounds as a source of energy by taking electrons from the reduced substrate and transferring them to a terminal electron acceptor in a redox reaction. This reaction releases energy that can be used to synthesise ATP and drive metabolism. In aerobic organisms, oxygen is used as the electron acceptor. In anaerobic organisms other inorganic compounds, such as nitrate, sulfate or carbon dioxide are used as electron acceptors. This leads to the ecologically important processes of denitrification, sulfate reduction and acetogenesis, respectively.

Another way of life of chemotrophs in the absence of possible electron acceptors is fermentation, where the electrons taken from the reduced substrates are transferred to oxidised intermediates to generate reduced fermentation products (e.g. lactate, ethanol, hydrogen, butyric acid). Fermentation is possible, because the energy content of the substrates is higher than that of the products, which allows the organisms to synthesise ATP and drive their metabolism. These processes are also important in biological responses to pollution; for example, sulfate-reducing bacteria are largely responsible for the production of the highly toxic forms of mercury (methyl- and dimethylmercury) in the environment. Non-respiratory anaerobes use fermentation to generate energy and reducing power, secreting metabolic by-products (such as ethanol in brewing) as waste. Facultative anaerobes can switch between fermentation and different terminal electron acceptors depending on the environmental conditions in which they find themselves.

Lithotrophic bacteria can use inorganic compounds as a source of energy. Common inorganic electron donors are hydrogen, carbon monoxide, ammonia (leading to nitrification), ferrous iron and other reduced metal ions, and several reduced sulphur compounds. Unusually, the gas methane can be used by methanotrophic bacteria as both a source of electrons and a substrate for carbon anabolism. In both aerobic phototrophy and chemolithotrophy, oxygen is used as a terminal electron acceptor, while under anaerobic conditions inorganic compounds are used instead. Most lithotrophic organisms are autotrophic, whereas organotrophic organisms are heterotrophic.

In addition to fixing carbon dioxide in photosynthesis, some bacteria also fix nitrogen gas (nitrogen fixation) using the enzyme nitrogenase. This environmentally important trait can be found in bacteria of nearly all the metabolic types listed above, but is not universal.

Growth and Reproduction

Unlike multicellular organisms, increases in the size of bacteria (cell growth) and their reproduction by cell division are tightly linked in unicellular organisms. Bacteria grow to a fixed size and then reproduce through binary fission, a form of asexual reproduction. Under optimal conditions, bacteria can grow and divide extremely rapidly, and bacterial populations can double as quickly as every 9.8 minutes. In cell division, two identical clone daughter cells are produced. Some bacteria, while still reproducing asexually, form more complex reproductive structures that help disperse the newly formed daughter cells. Examples include fruiting body formation by *Myxobacteria* and aerial hyphae formation by *Streptomyces*, or budding. Budding involves a cell forming a protrusion that breaks away and produces a daughter cell.

In the laboratory, bacteria are usually grown using solid or liquid media. Solid growth media such as agar plates are used to isolate pure cultures of a bacterial strain. However, liquid growth media are used when measurement of growth or large volumes of cells are required. Growth in stirred liquid media occurs as an even cell suspension, making the cultures easy to divide and transfer, although isolating single bacteria from liquid media is difficult. The use of selective media (media with specific nutrients added or deficient, or with antibiotics added) can help identify specific organisms.

Most laboratory techniques for growing bacteria use high levels of nutrients to produce large amounts of cells cheaply and quickly. However, in natural environments nutrients are limited, meaning that bacteria cannot continue to reproduce indefinitely. This nutrient limitation has led the evolution of different growth strategies. Some organisms can grow extremely rapidly when nutrients become available, such as the formation of algal (and cyanobacterial) blooms that often occur in lakes during the summer. Other organisms have adaptations to harsh environments, such as the production of multiple antibiotics by *Streptomyces* that inhibit the growth of competing microorganisms. In nature, many organisms live in communities (e.g. biofilms) which may allow for increased supply of nutrients and protection from environmental stresses. These relationships can be essential for growth of a particular organism or group of organisms (syntrophy).

Bacterial growth follows three phases. When a population of bacteria first enter a high-nutrient environment that allows growth, the cells need to adapt to their new environment. The first phase of growth is the lag phase, a period of slow growth when the cells are adapting to the high-nutrient environment and preparing for fast growth. The lag phase has high biosynthesis rates, as proteins necessary for rapid growth are produced. The second phase of growth is the logarithmic phase (log phase), also known as the exponential phase.

The log phase is marked by rapid exponential growth. The rate at which cells grow during this phase is known as the *growth rate* (*k*), and the time it takes the cells to double is known as the *generation time* (*g*). During log phase, nutrients are metabolised at maximum speed until one of the nutrients is depleted and starts limiting growth. The final phase of growth is the *stationary phase* and is caused by depleted nutrients.

The cells reduce their metabolic activity and consume non-essential cellular proteins. The stationary phase is a transition from rapid growth to a stress response state and there is increased expression of genes involved in DNA repair, antioxidant metabolism and nutrient transport.

Genetics

Most bacteria have a single circular chromosome that can range in size from only 160,000 base pairs in the endosymbiotic bacteria *Candidatus Carsonella ruddii*, to 12,200,000 base pairs in the soil-dwelling bacteria *Sorangium cellulosum*. Spirochaetes of the genus *Borrelia* are a notable exception to this arrangement, with bacteria such as *Borrelia burgdorferi*, the cause of Lyme disease, containing a single linear chromosome. The genes in bacterial genomes are usually a single continuous stretch of DNA and although several different types of introns do exist in bacteria, these are much more rare than in eukaryotes.

Bacteria may also contain plasmids, which are small extra-chromosomal DNAs that may contain genes for antibiotic resistance or virulence factors. Bacteria, as asexual organisms, inherit identical copies of their parent's genes (i.e., they are clonal). However, all bacteria can evolve by selection on changes to their genetic material DNA caused by genetic recombination or mutations. Mutations come from errors made during the replication of DNA or from exposure to mutagens. Mutation rates vary widely among different species of bacteria and even among different clones of a single species of bacteria. Genetic changes in bacterial genomes come from either random mutation during replication or "stress-directed mutation", where genes involved in a particular growth-limiting process have an increased mutation rate.

Some bacteria also transfer genetic material between cells. This can occur in three main ways. Firstly, bacteria can take up exogenous DNA from their environment, in a process called transformation. Genes can also be transferred by the process of transduction, when the integration of a bacteriophage introduces foreign DNA into the chromosome. The third method of gene transfer is bacterial conjugation, where DNA is transferred through direct cell contact. This gene acquisition from other bacteria or the environment is called horizontal gene transfer and may be common under natural conditions. Gene transfer is particularly important in antibiotic resistance as it allows the rapid transfer of resistance genes between different pathogens.

Bacteriophages

Bacteriophages are viruses that infect bacteria. Many types of bacteriophage exist, some simply infect and lyse their host bacteria, while others insert into the bacterial chromosome. A bacteriophage can contain genes that contribute to its host's phenotype: for example, in the evolution of *Escherichia coli* O157:H7 and *Clostridium botulinum*, the toxin genes in an integrated phage converted a harmless ancestral bacterium into a lethal pathogen. Bacteria resist phage infection through restriction modification systems that degrade foreign DNA, and a system that uses CRISPR sequences to retain fragments of the genomes of phage that the bacteria have come into contact with in the past, which allows them to block virus replication through a form of RNA interference. This CRISPR system provides bacteria with acquired immunity to infection.

Behaviour

Secretion : Bacteria frequently secrete chemicals into their environment in order to modify it favorably. The secretions are often proteins and may act as enzymes that digest some form of food in the environment.

Bioluminescence : A few bacteria have chemical systems that generate light. This bioluminescence often occurs in bacteria that live in association with fish, and the light probably serves to attract fish or other large animals.

Multicellularity : Bacteria often function as multicellular aggregates known as biofilms, exchanging a variety of molecular signals for inter-cell communication, and engaging in coordinated multicellular behaviour. The communal benefits of multicellular cooperation include a cellular division of labour, accessing resources that cannot effectively be utilized by single cells, collectively defending against antagonists, and optimizing population survival by differentiating into distinct cell types. For example, bacteria in biofilms can have more than 500 times increased resistance to antibacterial agents than individual "planktonic" bacteria of the same species.

One type of inter-cellular communication by a molecular signal is called quorum sensing, which serves the purpose of determining whether there is a local population density that is sufficiently high that it is productive to invest in processes that are only successful if large numbers of similar organisms behave similarly, as in excreting digestive enzymes or emitting light. Quorum sensing allows bacteria to coordinate gene expression, and enables them to produce, release and detect autoinducers or pheromones which accumulate with the growth in cell population.

Movement : Many bacteria can move using a variety of mechanisms: flagella are used for swimming through water; bacterial gliding and twitching motility move bacteria across surfaces; and changes of buoyancy allow vertical motion.

Swimming bacteria frequently move near 10 body lengths per second and a few as fast as 100. This makes them at least as fast as fish, on a relative scale.

In twitching motility, bacterial use their type IV pili as a grappling hook, repeatedly extending it, anchoring it and then retracting it with remarkable force (>80 pN).

Flagella are semi-rigid cylindrical structures that are rotated and function much like the propeller on a ship. Objects as small as bacteria operate a low Reynolds number and cylindrical forms are more efficient than the flat, paddle-like, forms appropriate at human size scale.

Bacterial species differ in the number and arrangement of flagella on their surface; some have a single flagellum (monotrichous), a flagellum at each end (amphitrichous), clusters of flagella at the poles of the cell (lophotrichous), while others have flagella distributed over the entire surface of the cell (peritrichous). The bacterial flagella is the best-understood motility structure in any organism and is made of about 20 proteins, with approximately another 30 proteins required for its regulation and assembly. The flagellum is a rotating structure driven by a reversible motor at the base that uses the electrochemical gradient across the membrane for power. This motor drives the motion of the filament, which acts as a propeller.

Many bacteria (such as *E. coli*) have two distinct modes of movement: forward movement (swimming) and tumbling. The tumbling allows them to reorient and makes their movement a three-dimensional random walk. The flagella of a unique group of bacteria, the spirochaetes, are found between two membranes in the periplasmic space. They have a distinctive helical body that twists about as it moves. Motile bacteria are attracted or repelled by certain stimuli in behaviours called *taxes*: these include chemotaxis, phototaxis, energy taxis and magnetotaxis. In one peculiar group, the myxobacteria, individual bacteria move together to form waves of cells that then differentiate to form fruiting bodies containing spores. The myxobacteria move only when on solid surfaces, unlike *E. coli* which is motile in liquid or solid media.

Several *Listeria* and *Shigella* species move inside host cells by usurping the cytoskeleton, which is normally used to move organelles inside the cell. By promoting actin polymerization at one pole of their cells, they can form a kind of tail that pushes them through the host cell's cytoplasm.

Classification and Identification

Classification seeks to describe the diversity of bacterial species by naming and grouping organisms based on similarities. Bacteria can be classified on the basis of cell structure, cellular metabolism or on differences in cell components such as DNA, fatty acids, pigments, antigens and quinones. While these schemes allowed the identification and classification of bacterial strains, it was unclear whether these differences represented variation between distinct species or between strains of the same species. This uncertainty was due to the lack of distinctive structures in most bacteria, as well as lateral gene transfer between unrelated species. Due to lateral gene transfer, some closely related bacteria can have very different morphologies and metabolisms.

To overcome this uncertainty, modern bacterial classification emphasizes molecular systematics, using genetic techniques such as guanine cytosine ratio determination, genome-genome hybridization, as well as sequencing genes that have not undergone extensive lateral gene transfer, such as the rRNA gene. Classification of bacteria is determined by publication in the International Journal of Systematic Bacteriology, and Bergey's Manual of Systematic Bacteriology. The International Committee on Systematic Bacteriology (ICSB) maintains international rules for the naming of bacteria and taxonomic categories and for the ranking of them in the International Code of Nomenclature of Bacteria.

The term "bacteria" was traditionally applied to all microscopic, single-celled prokaryotes. However, molecular systematics showed prokaryotic life to consist of two separate domains, originally called *Eubacteria* and *Archaebacteria*, but now called *Bacteria* and *Archaea* that evolved independently from an ancient common ancestor. The archaea and eukaryotes are more closely related to each other than either is to the bacteria. These two domains, along with Eukarya, are the basis of the three-domain system, which is currently the most widely used classification system in microbiolology. However, due to the relatively recent introduction of molecular systematics and a rapid increase in the number of genome sequences that are available, bacterial classification remains a changing and expanding field. For example, a few biologists argue that the Archaea and Eukaryotes evolved from Gram-positive bacteria.

Identification of bacteria in the laboratory is particularly relevant in medicine, where the correct treatment is determined by the bacterial species causing an infection. Consequently, the need to identify human pathogens was a major impetus for the development of techniques to identify bacteria.

The Gram stain, developed in 1884 by Hans Christian Gram, characterises bacteria based on the structural characteristics of their cell walls. The thick layers of peptidoglycan in the "Gram-positive" cell wall stain purple, while the thin "Gram-negative" cell wall appears pink. By combining morphology and Gram-staining, most bacteria can be classified as belonging to one of four groups (Gram-positive cocci, Gram-positive bacilli, Gram-negative cocci and Gram-negative bacilli). Some organisms are best identified by stains other than the Gram stain, particularly mycobacteria or *Nocardia*, which show acid-fastness on Ziehl–Neelsen or similar stains. Other organisms may need to be identified by their growth in special media, or by other techniques, such as serology. Culture techniques are designed to promote the growth and identify particular bacteria, while restricting the growth of the other bacteria in the sample. Often these techniques are designed for specific specimens; for example, a sputum sample will be treated to identify organisms that cause pneumonia, while stool specimens are cultured on selective media to identify organisms that cause diarrhoea, while preventing growth of non-pathogenic bacteria. Specimens that are normally sterile, such as blood, urine or spinal fluid, are cultured under conditions designed to grow all possible organisms. Once a pathogenic organism has been isolated, it can be further characterised by its morphology, growth patterns such as (aerobic or anaerobic growth, patterns of hemolysis) and staining. As with bacterial classification, identification of bacteria is increasingly using molecular methods. Diagnostics using such DNA-based tools, such as polymerase chain reaction, are increasingly popular due to their specificity and speed, compared to culture-based methods. These methods also allow the detection and identification of "viable but nonculturable" cells that are metabolically active but non-dividing.

However, even using these improved methods, the total number of bacterial species is not known and cannot even be estimated with any certainty. Following present classification, there are fewer than 9,000 known species of bacteria (including cyanobacteria), but attempts to estimate the true level of bacterial diversity have ranged from 10^7 to 10^9 total species – and even these diverse estimates may be off by many orders of magnitude.

Interactions with other Organisms

Despite their apparent simplicity, bacteria can form complex associations with other organisms. These symbiotic associations can be divided into parasitism, mutualism and commensalism. Due to their small size, commensal bacteria are ubiquitous and grow on animals and plants exactly as they will grow on any other surface. However, their growth can be increased by warmth and sweat, and large populations of these organisms in humans are the cause of body odor.

Predators

Some species of bacteria kill and then consume other microorganisms, these species called *predatory bacteria*. These include organisms such as *Myxococcus xanthus*, which forms swarms of cells that kill and digest any bacteria they encounter. Other bacterial predators either attach to their prey in order to digest them and absorb nutrients, such as *Vampirococcus*, or invade another cell and multiply inside the cytosol, such as *Daptobacter*. These predatory bacteria are thought to have evolved from saprophages that consumed dead microorganisms, through adaptations that allowed them to entrap and kill other organisms.

Mutualists

Certain bacteria form close spatial associations that are essential for their survival. One such mutualistic association, called interspecies hydrogen transfer, occurs between clusters of anaerobic bacteria that consume organic acids such as butyric acid or propionic acid and produce hydrogen, and methanogenic Archaea that consume hydrogen. The bacteria in this association are unable to consume the organic acids as this reaction produces hydrogen that accumulates in their surroundings. Only the intimate association with the hydrogen-consuming Archaea keeps the hydrogen concentration low enough to allow the bacteria to grow. In soil, microorganisms which reside in the rhizosphere (a zone that includes the root surface and the soil that adheres to the root after gentle shaking) carry out nitrogen fixation, converting nitrogen gas to nitrogenous compounds. This serves to provide an easily absorbable form of nitrogen for many plants, which cannot fix nitrogen themselves. Many other bacteria are found as symbionts in humans and other organisms. For example, the presence of over 1,000 bacterial species in the normal human gut flora of the intestines can contribute to gut immunity, synthesise vitamins such as folic acid, vitamin K and biotin, convert milk protein to lactic acid, as well as fermenting complex undigestible carbohydrates. The presence of this gut flora also inhibits the growth of potentially pathogenic bacteria (usually through competitive exclusion) and these beneficial bacteria are consequently sold as probiotic dietary supplements.

Pathogens

If bacteria form a parasitic association with other organisms, they are classed as pathogens. Pathogenic bacteria are a major cause of human death and disease and cause infections such as tetanus, typhoid fever, diphtheria, syphilis, cholera, foodborne illness, leprosy and tuberculosis. A pathogenic cause for a known medical disease may only be discovered many years after, as was the case with *Helicobacter pylori* and peptic ulcer disease. Bacterial diseases are also important in agriculture, with bacteria causing leaf spot, fire blight and wilts in plants, as well as Johne's disease, mastitis, salmonella and anthrax in farm animals.

Each species of pathogen has a characteristic spectrum of interactions with its human hosts. Some organisms, such as *Staphylococcus* or *Streptococcus*, can cause skin infections, pneumonia, meningitis and even overwhelming sepsis, a systemic inflammatory response producing shock, massive vasodilation and death. Yet these organisms are also part of the normal human flora and usually exist on the skin or in the nose without causing any disease at all.

Other organisms invariably cause disease in humans, such as the Rickettsia, which are obligate intracellular parasites able to grow and reproduce only within the cells of other organisms. One species of Rickettsia causes typhus, while another causes Rocky Mountain spotted fever. *Chlamydia*, another phylum of obligate intracellular parasites, contains species that can cause pneumonia, or urinary tract infection and may be involved in coronary heart disease. Finally, some species such as *Pseudomonas aeruginosa*, *Burkholderia cenocepacia*, and *Mycobacterium avium* are opportunistic pathogens and cause disease mainly in people suffering from immunosuppression or cystic fibrosis.

Bacterial infections may be treated with antibiotics, which are classified as bacteriocidal if they kill bacteria, or bacteriostatic if they just prevent bacterial growth. There are many types of antibiotics and each class inhibits a process that is different in the pathogen from that found in the host. An example of how antibiotics produce selective toxicity are chloramphenicol and puromycin, which inhibit the bacterial ribosome, but not the structurally different eukaryotic ribosome.

Antibiotics are used both in treating human disease and in intensive farming to promote animal growth, where they may be contributing to the rapid development of antibiotic resistance in bacterial populations. Infections can be prevented by antiseptic measures such as sterilizating the skin prior to piercing it with the needle of a syringe, and by proper care of indwelling catheters. Surgical and dental instruments are also sterilized to prevent contamination by bacteria. Disinfectants such as bleach are used to kill bacteria or other pathogens on surfaces to prevent contamination and further reduce the risk of infection.

Significance in Technology and Industry

Bacteria, often lactic acid bacteria such as *Lactobacillus* and *Lactococcus*, in combination with yeasts and molds, have been used for thousands of years in the preparation of fermented foods such as cheese, pickles, soy sauce, sauerkraut, vinegar, wine and yoghurt.

The ability of bacteria to degrade a variety of organic compounds is remarkable and has been used in waste processing and bioremediation. Bacteria capable of digesting the hydrocarbons in petroleum are often used to clean up oil spills. Fertilizer was added to some of the beaches in Prince William Sound in an attempt to promote the growth of these naturally occurring bacteria after the infamous 1989 *Exxon Valdez* oil spill. These efforts were effective on beaches that were not too thickly covered in oil. Bacteria are also used for the bioremediation of industrial toxic wastes. In the chemical industry, bacteria are most important in the production of enantiomerically pure chemicals for use as pharmaceuticals or agrichemicals.

Bacteria can also be used in the place of pesticides in the biological pest control. This commonly involves *Bacillus thuringiensis* (also called BT), a Gram-positive, soil dwelling bacterium. Subspecies of this bacteria are used as a Lepidopteran-specific insecticides under trade names such as Dipel and Thuricide. Because of their specificity, these pesticides are regarded as environmentally friendly, with little or no effect on humans, wildlife, pollinators and most other beneficial insects. Because of their ability to quickly grow and the relative ease with which they can be manipulated, bacteria are the workhorses for the fields of molecular biology, genetics and biochemistry. By making mutations in bacterial DNA and examining the resulting phenotypes, scientists can determine the function of genes, enzymes and metabolic pathways in bacteria, then apply this knowledge to more complex organisms. This aim of understanding the biochemistry of a cell reaches its most complex expression in the synthesis of huge amounts of enzyme kinetic and gene expression data into mathematical models of entire organisms. This is achievable in some well-studied bacteria, with models of *Escherichia coli* metabolism now being produced and tested. This understanding of bacterial metabolism and genetics allows the use of biotechnology to bioengineer bacteria for the production of therapeutic proteins, such as insulin, growth factors, or antibodies.

Classification of Pathogenic Bacteria

Pathogenic bacteria are bacteria that cause bacterial infection. This article deals with human pathogenic bacteria.

Although the vast majority of bacteria are harmless or beneficial, quite a few bacteria are pathogenic. One of the bacterial diseases with highest disease burden is tuberculosis, caused by the bacterium *Mycobacterium tuberculosis*, which kills about 2 million people a year, mostly in sub-Saharan Africa. Pathogenic bacteria contribute to other globally important diseases, such as pneumonia, which can be caused by bacteria such as *Streptococcus* and *Pseudomonas*, and foodborne illnesses, which can be caused by bacteria such as *Shigella*, *Campylobacter* and *Salmonella*. Pathogenic bacteria also cause infections such as tetanus, typhoid fever, diphtheria, syphilis and leprosy.

Koch's postulates are criteria designed to establish a causal relationship between a causative microbe and a disease.

Diseases

Each pathogenic species has a characteristic spectrum of interactions with its human hosts.

Conditionally Pathogenic

Conditionally pathogenic bacteria are only pathogenic under certain conditions, such as a wound that allows for entry into the blood, or a decrease in immune function. For example, *Staphylococcus* or *Streptococcus* are also part of the normal human flora and usually exist on the skin or in the nose without causing disease, but can potentially cause skin infections, pneumonia, meningitis and even overwhelming sepsis, a systemic inflammatory response producing shock, massive vasodilation and death. Some species of bacteria, such as *Pseudomonas aeruginosa*, *Burkholderia cenocepacia*, and *Mycobacterium avium*, are opportunistic pathogens and cause disease mainly in people suffering from immunosuppression or cystic fibrosis.

Intracellular

Other organisms invariably cause disease in humans, such as obligate intracellular parasites that are able to grow and reproduce only within the cells of other organisms. Still, infections with intracellular bacteria may be asymptomatic, such as during the incubation period. An example of intracellular bacteria is *Rickettsia*. One species of *Rickettsia* causes typhus, while another causes Rocky Mountain spotted fever. Chlamydia, another phylum of obligate intracellular parasites, contains species that can cause pneumonia, or urinary tract infection and may be involved in coronary heart disease. *Mycobacterium* and *Brucella* can exist intracellularly, though they are facultative (not obligate intracellular parasites.)

Treatment

Bacterial infections may be treated with antibiotics, which are classified as bacteriocidal if they kill bacteria, or bacteriostatic if they just prevent bacterial growth. There are many types of antibiotics and each class inhibits a process that is different in the pathogen from that found in the host. For example, the antibiotics chloramphenicol and tetracyclin inhibit the bacterial ribosome, but not the structurally-different eukaryotic ribosome, and so exhibit selective toxicity. Antibiotics are used both in treating human disease and in intensive farming to promote animal growth. Both uses may be contributing to the rapid development of antibiotic resistance in bacterial populations. Infections can be prevented by antiseptic measures such as sterilizing the skin prior to piercing it with the needle of a syringe, and by proper care of indwelling catheters.

Surgical and dental instruments are also sterilized to prevent infection by bacteria. Disinfectants such as bleach are used to kill bacteria or other pathogens on surfaces to prevent contamination and further reduce the risk of infection. Most bacteria in food are killed by cooking to temperatures above 73 °C (163°F).

Staphylococcal Infections

Staphylococcus is a genus of Gram-positive bacteria which includes several species that can cause a wide variety of infections in humans and other animals through either toxin production or invasion. Staphylococcal toxins are a common cause of food poisoning, as they can be produced in improperly-stored food.

Coagulase-positive

The main coagulase-positive Staphylococcus is *Staphylococcus aureus*. These bacteria can survive on dry surfaces, increasing the chance of transmission. *S. aureus* is also implicated in toxic shock syndrome; during the 1980s some tampons allowed the rapid growth of *S. aureus*, which released toxins that were absorbed into the bloodstream. Any *S. aureus* infection can cause the staphylococcal scalded skin syndrome, a cutaneous reaction to exotoxin absorbed into the bloodstream. It can also cause a type of septicaemia called pyaemia. The infection can be life-threatening. Problematically, Methicillin-resistant *Staphylococcus aureus* has become a major cause of hospital-acquired infections, and is being recognized with increasing frequency in community-acquired infections.

Etymology

The term Staphylococcus is derived from the Greek word "staphyle" meaning a bunch of grapes, and "kokkos" means berries. The bacteria, when seen under a microscope appear like a branch of grapes or berries.

Main Staphylococcus aureus Infections

Type	*Examples*
Localized skin infections	• Stye and other small, superficial abscesses in sweat or sebaceous glands • Subcutaneous abscesses (boils) around foreign bodies • Large, deep, infections (carbuncles) possibly causing bacteremia
Diffuse skin infection	• Impetigo
Deep, localized infections	• Acute and chronic osteomyelitis • Septic arthritis

Contd...

Type	*Examples*
Other infections	• Acute infective endocarditis • Septicemia • Necrotizing pneumonia
Toxinoses	• Toxic shock syndrome • Gastroenteritis • Scalded skin syndrome.

Other infections include:

- Closed-space infections of the fingertips, known as paronychia.

Coagulase-negative

- *S. epidermidis*, a coagulase-negative staphylococcus species, is a commensal of the skin, but can cause severe infections in immune-suppressed patients and those with central venous catheters.
- *S. saprophyticus*, another coagulase-negative species that is part of the normal vaginal flora, is predominantly implicated in genitourinary tract infections in sexually-active young women.
- In recent years, several other *Staphylococcus* species have been implicated in human infections, notably *S. lugdunensis*, *S. schleiferi*, and *S. caprae*.

Streptococcal Infections

Streptococcus is a genus of spherical Gram-positive bacteria belonging to the phylum Firmicutes and the lactic acid bacteria group. Cellular division occurs along a single axis in these bacteria, and thus they grow in chains or pairs, hence the name — from Greek *streptos*, meaning easily bent or twisted, like a chain (twisted chain). Contrast this with staphylococci, which divide along multiple axes and generate grape-like clusters of cells. Streptococci are oxidase- and catalase-negative, and many are facultative anaerobes.

In 1984, many organisms formerly considered *Streptococcus* were separated out into the genera *Enterococcus* and *Lactococcus*.

Pathogenesis

In addition to streptococcal pharyngitis (or *strep throat*), certain *Streptococcus* species are responsible for many cases of meningitis, bacterial pneumonia, endocarditis, erysipelas and necrotizing fasciitis (the 'flesh-eating' bacterial infections). However, many streptococcal species are non-pathogenic.

Indeed, Streptococci are a necessary ingredient in Emmentaler ("Swiss") cheese. Streptococci are also part of the normal commensal flora of the mouth, skin, intestine, and upper respiratory tract of humans.

As a rule, individual species of *Streptococcus* are classified based on their hemolytic properties. Alpha hemolysis is caused by an oxidation of iron in hemoglobin, giving it a greenish color on blood agar. Beta-hemolysis is complete rupture of red blood cells, giving distinct, wide, clear areas around bacterial colonies on blood agar. Other streptococci are labelled as gamma hemolytic, actually a misnomer, as no hemolysis takes place.

Beta-hemolytic streptococci are further characterised via the Lancefield serotyping – based on specific carbohydrates in the bacterial cell wall. These are named Lancefield groups A to v (except I and J). In the medical setting, the most important groups are the alpha-hemolytic streptococci, *S. pneumoniae* and *Streptococcus* Viridans-group, and the beta-hemolytic streptococci of Lancefield groups A and B (also known as "Group A strep" and "Group B strep").

Alpha-hemolytic

Pneumococci

- *S. pneumoniae* (sometimes called Pneumococcus), a leading cause of bacterial pneumonia and occasional etiology of otitis media, sinusitis, meningitis and peritonitis.

The Viridans Group: Alpha Hemolytic

- *S. mutans*, a contributor to dental caries
- *S. mitis*, mostly found around cheek region
- *S. sanguinis*, no preference of locations
- *S. salivarius*, mostly found on the dorsal side of the tongue
- *S. salivarius ssp. thermophilus*, used in the manufacture of some cheeses and yogurts
- *S. constellatus*, occasional human pathogen, notable as colonies grown on blood agar smell strongly of caramel.

Beta-hemolytic

Group A : *S. pyogenes*, also known as *Group A Streptococcus* (*GAS*), is the causative agent in Group A streptococcal infections, including streptococcal pharyngitis ("strep throat" AmE), acute rheumatic fever, scarlet fever, acute glomerulonephritis and necrotizing fasciitis. Other *Streptococcus* species may also possess the Group A antigen, but human infections by non-*S. pyogenes* GAS strains (some *S. dysgalactiae* subsp. *equisimilis* and *S. anginosus* Group strains) appear to be uncommon. Group A *Streptococcus* infection is generally diagnosed with a Rapid Strep Test (AmE) or by culture.

Rheumatic fever, a disease that affects the joints and heart valves, is a consequence of untreated strep A infection caused not by the bacterium itself. Rheumatic fever is caused by the antibodies created by the immune system to fight off the infection cross-reacting with other proteins in the body. This cross-reaction causes the body to essentially attack itself and leads to the damage above.

Group B : *S. agalactiae*, or *GBS*, causes pneumonia and meningitis in neonates and the elderly, with occasional systemic bacteremia. They can also colonize the intestines and the female reproductive tract, increasing the risk for premature rupture of membranes and transmission to the infant. The American College of Obstetricians and Gynecologists, American Academy of Pediatrics and the Centers for Disease Control recommend all pregnant women between 35 and 37 weeks gestation should be tested for GBS. Women who test positive should be given prophylactic antibiotics during labour, which will usually prevent transmission to the infant. In the UK, clinicians have been slow to implement the same standards as the US, Australia and Canada.

In the UK, only 1% of maternity units test for the presence of Group B Streptococcus. Although The Royal College of Obstetricians and Gynaecologists issued risk-based guidelines in 2003 (due for review 2006), the implementation of these guidelines has been patchy. Some groups feel that as a result over 75 infants in the UK die each year of GBS related disease and another 600 or so suffer serious infection, most of which could be prevented however this is yet to be substantiated by randomized controlled trial in the UK setting and, given the evidence for the efficacy of testing and treating from other countries, it may be that the large-scale trial necessary would receive neither funding nor ethics approval.

Group C : Includes *S. equi*, which causes strangles in horses, and *S. zooepidemicus* - S. equi is a clonal descendent or biovar of the ancestral S. zooepidemicus - which causes infections in several species of mammals including cattle and horses.

The Group D strains include *Streptococcus bovis* and *Streptococcus equinus*.

Group G Streptococci

These streptococci are usually but not exclusively beta hemolytic. *Streptococcus canis* is an example of a GGS which is typically found on animals but can cause infection in humans.

Non-hemolytic

Group D (enterococci) : Many former Group D streptococci have been reclassified and placed in the genus *Enterococcus* (including *S. faecalis*, *S. faecium*, *S. durans*, and *S. avium*). For example, *Streptococcus faecalis* is now *Enterococcus faecalis*.

The remaining non-enterococcal Group D strains include *Streptococcus bovis* and *Streptococcus equinus*.

Non-hemolytic streptococci rarely cause illness. However, weakly hemolytic group D beta-hemolytic streptococci and *Listeria monocytogenes* (which is actually a gram positive bacillus) should not be confused with non-hemolytic streptococci.

Dental Caries

Dental caries, also known as tooth decay or a cavity, is a disease where bacterial processes damage hard tooth structure (enamel, dentin, and cementum). These tissues progressively break down, producing dental caries (cavities, holes in the teeth). Two groups of bacteria are responsible for initiating caries: *Streptococcus mutans* and *Lactobacillus*. If left untreated, the disease can lead to pain, tooth loss, infection, and, in severe cases, death. Today, caries remains one of the most common diseases throughout the world. Cariology is the study of dental caries.

The presentation of caries is highly variable; however, the risk factors and stages of development are similar. Initially, it may appear as a small chalky area that may eventually develop into a large cavitation. Sometimes caries may be directly visible, however other methods of detection such as radiographs are used for less visible areas of teeth and to judge the extent of destruction.

Tooth decay is caused by specific types of acid-producing bacteria that cause damage in the presence of fermentable carbohydrates such as sucrose, fructose, and glucose. The mineral content of teeth is sensitive to increases in acidity from the production of lactic acid. Specifically, a tooth (which is primarily mineral in content) is in a constant state of back-and-forth demineralization and remineralization between the tooth and surrounding saliva. When the pH at the surface of the tooth drops below 5.5, demineralization proceeds faster than remineralization (meaning that there is a net loss of mineral structure on the tooth's surface). This results in the ensuing decay. Depending on the extent of tooth destruction, various treatments can be used to restore teeth to proper form, function, and aesthetics, but there is no known method to regenerate large amounts of tooth structure, though stem cell related research suggests one possibility. Instead, dental health organizations advocate preventive and prophylactic measures, such as regular oral hygiene and dietary modifications, to avoid dental caries.

Classification

Caries can be classified by location, etiology, rate of progression, and affected hard tissues. These forms of classification can be used to characterize a particular case of tooth decay in order to more accurately represent the condition to others and also indicate the severity of tooth destruction.

Location

Generally, there are two types of caries when separated by location: caries found on smooth surfaces and caries found in pits and fissures. The location, development, and progression of smooth-surface caries differ from those of pit and fissure caries. G.V. Black created a classification system that is widely used and based on the location of the caries on the tooth. The original classification distinguished caries into five groups, indicated by the word "Class", and a Roman numeral. Pit and fissure caries is indicated as Class I; smooth surface caries is further divided into Class II, Class III, Class IV, and Class V. A Class VI was added onto Black's Classification of Caries Lesions and also represents a smooth-surface carious lesion.

Pit and Fissure Caries (Class I Dental Caries)

Pits and fissures are anatomic landmarks on a tooth where the enamel folds inward. Fissures are formed during the development of grooves but the enamel in the area is not fully fused. As a result, a deep linear depression forms in the enamel's surface structure, which forms a location for dental caries to develop and flourish. Fissures are mostly located on the occlusal (chewing) surfaces of posterior (rear) teeth and palatal surfaces of maxillary anterior (front) teeth. Pits are small, pinpoint depressions that are most commonly found at the ends or cross-sections of grooves. In particular, buccal pits are found on the facial surfaces of molars. For all types of pits and fissures, the deep infolding of enamel makes oral hygiene along these surfaces difficult, allowing dental caries to develop more commonly in these areas.

The occlusal surfaces of teeth represent 12.5% of all tooth surfaces but are the location of over 50% of all dental caries. Among children, pit and fissure caries represent 90% of all dental caries. Pit and fissure caries can sometimes be difficult to detect. As the decay progresses, caries in enamel nearest the surface of the tooth spreads gradually deeper. Once the caries reaches the dentin at the dentino-enamel junction (DEJ), the decay quickly spreads laterally. Within the dentin, the decay follows a triangle pattern that points to the tooth's pulp. This pattern of decay is typically described as two triangles (one triangle in enamel, and another in dentin) with their bases conjoined to each other at the DEJ. This base-to-base pattern is typical of pit and fissure caries, unlike smooth-surface caries (where base and apex of the two triangles join).

Smooth-surface Caries

There are three types of smooth-surface caries. Proximal caries, also called interproximal caries, form on the smooth surfaces between adjacent teeth. Root caries form on the root surfaces of teeth. The third type of smooth-surface caries occur on any other smooth tooth surface. Proximal caries are the most difficult type to detect. Frequently, this type of caries cannot be detected visually or manually with a dental explorer. Proximal caries form cervically (toward the roots of a tooth) just under the contact between two teeth. As a result, radiographs are needed for early discovery of proximal caries. Under Black's classification system, proximal caries on posterior teeth (premolars and molars) are designated as Class II caries. Proximal caries on anterior teeth (incisors and canines) are indicated as Class III if the incisal edge (chewing surface) is not included and Class IV if the incisal edge is included.

Root caries, which are sometimes described as a category of smooth-surfaces caries, are the third most common type of caries and usually occur when the root surfaces have been exposed due to gingival recession. When the gingiva is healthy, root caries is unlikely to develop because the root surfaces are not as accessible to bacterial plaque. The root surface is more vulnerable to the demineralization process than enamel because cementum begins to demineralize at 6.7 pH, which is higher than enamel's critical pH. Regardless, it is easier to arrest the progression of root caries than enamel caries because roots have a greater reuptake of fluoride than enamel. Root caries are most likely to be found on facial surfaces, then interproximal surfaces, then lingual surfaces. Mandibular molars are the most common location to find root caries, followed by mandibular premolars, maxillary anteriors, maxillary posteriors, and mandibular anteriors.

Lesions on other smooth surfaces of teeth are also possible. Since these occur in all smooth surface areas of enamel except for interproximal areas, these types of caries are easily detected and are associated with high levels of plaque and diets promoting caries formation. Under Black's classification system, caries near the gingiva on the facial or lingual surfaces is designated Class V. Class VI is reserved for caries confined to cusp tips on posterior teeth or incisal edges of anterior teeth.

Other General Descriptions

Besides the two previously mentioned categories, carious lesions can be described further by their location on a particular surface of a tooth. Caries on a tooth's surface that are nearest the cheeks or lips are called "facial caries", and caries on surfaces facing the tongue are known as "lingual caries".

Facial caries can be subdivided into buccal (when found on the surfaces of posterior teeth nearest the cheeks) and labial (when found on the surfaces of anterior teeth nearest the lips). Lingual caries can also be described as palatal when found on the lingual surfaces of maxillary teeth because they are located beside the hard palate.

Caries near a tooth's cervix—the location where the crown of a tooth and its roots meet—are referred to as cervical caries. Occlusal caries are found on the chewing surfaces of posterior teeth. Incisal caries are caries found on the chewing surfaces of anterior teeth.

Caries can also be described as "mesial" or "distal." Mesial signifies a location on a tooth closer to the median line of the face, which is located on a vertical axis between the eyes, down the nose, and between the contact of the central incisors. Locations on a tooth further away from the median line are described as distal.

Etiology

In some instances, caries are described in other ways that might indicate the cause. "Baby bottle caries", "early childhood caries", or "baby bottle tooth decay" is a pattern of decay found in young children with their deciduous (baby) teeth. The teeth most likely affected are the maxillary anterior teeth, but all teeth can be affected.

The name for this type of caries comes from the fact that the decay usually is a result of allowing children to fall asleep with sweetened liquids in their bottles or feeding children sweetened liquids multiple times during the day. Another pattern of decay is “rampant caries”, which signifies advanced or severe decay on multiple surfaces of many teeth. Rampant caries may be seen in individuals with xerostomia, poor oral hygiene, stimulant use (due to drug-induced dry mouth), and/or large sugar intake. If rampant caries is a result of previous radiation to the head and neck, it may be described as radiation-induced caries. Problems can also be caused by the self destruction of roots and whole tooth resorption when new teeth erupt or later from unknown causes. Dr. Miller stated in 1887 that “Dental decay is chemico-parasitic process consisting of two stages, the decalcification of enamel, which results in its total destruction and the decalcification of dentin as a preliminary stage followed by dissolution of the softened residue.” In his hypothesis, Dr.Miller assigned essential roles to three factors:

1. Carbohydrate substrate.
2. Acid which caused dissolution of tooth minerals.
3. Oral micro organisms which produce acid and also cause proteolysis.

Rate of Progression

Temporal descriptions can be applied to caries to indicate the progression rate and previous history. “Acute” signifies a quickly developing condition, whereas “chronic” describes a condition which has taken an extended time to develop where thousands of meals and snacks, many causing some acid demineralisation that is not remineralized and eventually results in cavities. Fluoride treatment can help recalcification of tooth enamel. Recurrent caries, also described as secondary, are caries that appears at a location with a previous history of caries. This is frequently found on the margins of fillings and other dental restorations. On the other hand, incipient caries describes decay at a location that has not experienced previous decay. Arrested caries describes a lesion on a tooth which was previously demineralized but was remineralized before causing a cavitation. Using fluoride treatments can help with recalcification.

Affected Hard Tissue

Depending on which hard tissues are affected, it is possible to describe caries as involving enamel, dentin, or cementum. Early in its development, caries may affect only enamel. Once the extent of decay reaches the deeper layer of dentin, "dentinal caries" is used. Since cementum is the hard tissue that covers the roots of teeth, it is not often affected by decay unless the roots of teeth are exposed to the mouth. Although the term "cementum caries" may be used to describe the decay on roots of teeth, very rarely does caries affect the cementum alone. Roots have a very thin layer of cementum over a large layer of dentin, and thus most caries affecting cementum also affects dentin.

Signs and Symptoms

A person experiencing caries may not be aware of the disease. The earliest sign of a new carious lesion is the appearance of a chalky white spot on the surface of the tooth, indicating an area of demineralization of enamel. This is referred to as incipient decay. As the lesion continues to demineralize, it can turn brown but will eventually turn into a cavitation ("cavity"). Before the cavity forms, the process is reversible, but once a cavity forms, the lost tooth structure cannot be regenerated. A lesion which appears brown and shiny suggests dental caries were once present but the demineralization process has stopped, leaving a stain. A brown spot which is dull in appearance is probably a sign of active caries. As the enamel and dentin are destroyed, the cavity becomes more noticeable. The affected areas of the tooth change color and become soft to the touch. Once the decay passes through enamel, the dentinal tubules, which have passages to the nerve of the tooth, become exposed and causes pain in the tooth. The pain may worsen with exposure to heat, cold, or sweet foods and drinks. Dental caries can also cause bad breath and foul tastes. In highly progressed cases, infection can spread from the tooth to the surrounding soft tissues. Complications such as cavernous sinus thrombosis and Ludwig's angina can be life-threatening.

Causes

There are four main criteria required for caries formation: a tooth surface (enamel or dentin); caries-causing bacteria; fermentable carbohydrates (such as sucrose); and time. The caries process does not have an inevitable outcome, and different individuals will be susceptible to different degrees depending on the shape of their teeth, oral hygiene habits, and the buffering capacity of their saliva. Dental caries can occur on any surface of a tooth which is exposed to the oral cavity, but not the structures which are retained within the bone.

Teeth

There are certain diseases and disorders affecting teeth which may leave an individual at a greater risk for caries. Amelogenesis imperfecta, which occurs between 1 in 718 and 1 in 14,000 individuals, is a disease in which the enamel does not fully form or forms in insufficient amounts and can fall off a tooth. In both cases, teeth may be left more vulnerable to decay because the enamel is not able to protect the tooth.

In most people, disorders or diseases affecting teeth are not the primary cause of dental caries. Ninety-six percent of tooth enamel is composed of minerals. These minerals, especially hydroxyapatite, will become soluble when exposed to acidic environments. Enamel begins to demineralize at a pH of 5.5. Dentin and cementum are more susceptible to caries than enamel because they have lower mineral content. Thus, when root surfaces of teeth are exposed from gingival recession or periodontal disease, caries can develop more readily. Even in a healthy oral environment, however, the tooth is susceptible to dental caries.

The anatomy of teeth may affect the likelihood of caries formation. Where the deep grooves of teeth are more numerous and exaggerated, pit and fissure caries are more likely to develop. Also, caries are more likely to develop when food is trapped between teeth.

Bacteria

The mouth contains a wide variety of oral bacteria, but only a few specific species of bacteria are believed to cause dental caries: *Streptococcus mutans* and *Lactobacilli* among them. *Lactobacillus acidophilus*, *Actinomyces viscosus*, *Nocardia spp.*, and *Streptococcus mutans* are most closely associated with caries, particularly root caries. Bacteria collect around the teeth and gums in a sticky, creamy-coloured mass called plaque, which serves as a biofilm. Some sites collect plaque more commonly than others. The grooves on the biting surfaces of molar and premolar teeth provide microscopic retention, as does the point of contact between teeth. Plaque may also collect along the gingiva.

Fermentable Carbohydrates

Bacteria in a person's mouth convert glucose, fructose, and most commonly sucrose into acids such as lactic acid through a glycolytic process called fermentation. If left in contact with the tooth, these acids may cause demineralization, which is the dissolution of its mineral content. The process is dynamic, however, as remineralization can also occur if the acid is neutralized by saliva or mouthwash. Fluoride toothpaste or dental varnish may aid remineralization. If demineralization continues over time, enough mineral content may be lost so that the soft organic material left behind disintegrates, forming a cavity or hole.

The impact such sugars have on the progress of dental caries is called cariogenicity. Sucrose, although a bound glucose and fructose unit, is in fact more cariogenic than a mixture of equal parts of glucose and fructose. This is due to the bacteria utilising the energy in the saccharide bond between the glucose and fructose subunits. *S.mutans* adheres to the biofilm on the tooth by converting sucrose into an extremely adhesive substance called dextran polysaccharide by the enzyme dextransucranase.

Time

The frequency of which teeth are exposed to cariogenic (acidic) environments affects the likelihood of caries development. After meals or snacks, the bacteria in the mouth metabolize sugar, resulting in an acidic by-product which decreases pH. As time progresses, the pH returns to normal due to the buffering capacity of saliva and the dissolved mineral content of tooth surfaces. During every exposure to the acidic environment, portions of the inorganic mineral content at the surface of teeth dissolves and can remain dissolved for two hours. Since teeth are vulnerable during these acidic periods, the development of dental caries relies heavily on the frequency of acid exposure.

The carious process can begin within days of a tooth erupting into the mouth if the diet is sufficiently rich in suitable carbohydrates. Evidence suggests that the introduction of fluoride treatments have slowed the process. Proximal caries take an average of four years to pass through enamel in permanent teeth. Because the cementum enveloping the root surface is not nearly as durable as the enamel encasing the crown, root caries tends to progress much more rapidly than decay on other surfaces.

The progression and loss of mineralization on the root surface is 2.5 times faster than caries in enamel. In very severe cases where oral hygiene is very poor and where the diet is very rich in fermentable carbohydrates, caries may cause cavities within months of tooth eruption. This can occur, for example, when children continuously drink sugary drinks from baby bottles.

Other Risk Factors

Reduced saliva is associated with increased caries since the buffering capability of saliva is not present to counterbalance the acidic environment created by certain foods. As result, medical conditions that reduce the amount of saliva produced by salivary glands, particularly the submandibular gland and parotid gland, are likely to lead to widespread tooth decay. Examples include Sjögren's syndrome, diabetes mellitus, diabetes insipidus, and sarcoidosis. Medications, such as antihistamines and antidepressants, can also impair salivary flow.

Stimulants, most notoriously methylamphetamine, also occlude the flow of saliva to an extreme degree. Abusers of stimulants tend to have poor oral hygiene. Tetrahydrocannabinol, the active chemical substance in cannabis, also causes a nearly complete occlusion of salivation, known colloquially as "cotton mouth". Moreover, sixty-three percent of the most commonly prescribed medications in the United States list dry mouth as a known side effect. Radiation therapy of the head and neck may also damage the cells in salivary glands, increasing the likelihood of caries formation. The use of tobacco may also increase the risk for caries formation. Some brands of smokeless tobacco contain high sugar content, increasing susceptibility to caries. Tobacco use is a significant risk factor for periodontal disease, which can cause the gingiva to recede. As the gingiva loses attachment to the teeth, the root surface becomes more visible in the mouth. If this occurs, root caries is a concern since the cementum covering the roots of teeth is more easily demineralized by acids than enamel. Currently, there is not enough evidence to support a causal relationship between smoking and coronal caries, but evidence does suggest a relationship between smoking and root-surface caries.

Intrauterine and neonatal lead exposure promote tooth decay. Besides lead, all atoms with electrical charge and ionic radius similar to bivalent calcium, such as cadmium, mimic the calcium ion and therefore exposure may promote tooth decay. Salivary and dietary iodine seems to play an important role in pathogenesis of dental caries and in salivary glands physiology. Saliva is rich in peroxidase enzymes and has high secretion of iodides. Iodine is able to penetrate directly through intact enamel in dentine, pulp and periodontal tissues and according to some researchers it is able to prevent some dental pathologies directly with antibacterial action, and also indirectly with an antioxidant mechanism.

Pathophysiology

Enamel: Enamel is a highly mineralized acellular tissue, and caries act upon it through a chemical process brought on by the acidic environment produced by bacteria. As the bacteria consume the sugar and use it for their own energy, they produce lactic acid. The effects of this process include the demineralization of crystals in the enamel, caused by acids, over time until the bacteria physically penetrate the dentin. Enamel rods, which are the basic unit of the enamel structure, run perpendicularly from the surface of the tooth to the dentin.

Since demineralization of enamel by caries generally follows the direction of the enamel rods, the different triangular patterns between pit and fissure and smooth-surface caries develop in the enamel because the orientation of enamel rods are different in the two areas of the tooth. As the enamel loses minerals, and dental caries progresses, the enamel develop several distinct zones, visible under a light microscope. From the deepest layer of the enamel to the enamel surface, the identified areas are the: translucent zone, dark zones, body of the lesion, and surface zone.

The translucent zone is the first visible sign of caries and coincides with a one to two percent loss of minerals. A slight remineralization of enamel occurs in the dark zone, which serves as an example of how the development of dental caries is an active process with alternating changes. The area of greatest demineralization and destruction is in the body of the lesion itself. The surface zone remains relatively mineralized and is present until the loss of tooth structure results in a cavitation.

Dentin: Unlike enamel, the dentin reacts to the progression of dental caries. After tooth formation, the ameloblasts, which produce enamel, are destroyed once enamel formation is complete and thus cannot later regenerate enamel after its destruction. On the other hand, dentin is produced continuously throughout life by odontoblasts, which reside at the border between the pulp and dentin. Since odontoblasts are present, a stimulus, such as caries, can trigger a biologic response.

These defense mechanisms include the formation of sclerotic and tertiary dentin. In dentin from the deepest layer to the enamel, the distinct areas affected by caries are the translucent zone, the zone of destruction, and the zone of bacterial penetration. The translucent zone represents the advancing front of the carious process and is where the initial demineralization begins. The zones of bacterial penetration and destruction are the locations of invading bacteria and ultimately the decomposition of dentin.

Sclerotic Dentin: The structure of dentin is an arrangement of microscopic channels, called dentinal tubules, which radiate outward from the pulp chamber to the exterior cementum or enamel border. The diameter of the dentinal tubules is largest near the pulp (about 2.5 ìm) and smallest (about 900 nm) at the junction of dentin and enamel.

The carious process continues through the dentinal tubules, which are responsible for the triangular patterns resulting from the progression of caries deep into the tooth. The tubules also allow caries to progress faster. In response, the fluid inside the tubules bring immunoglobulins from the immune system to fight the bacterial infection. At the same time, there is an increase of mineralization of the surrounding tubules.

This results in a constriction of the tubules, which is an attempt to slow the bacterial progression. In addition, as the acid from the bacteria demineralizes the hydroxyapatite crystals, calcium and phosphorus are released, allowing for the precipitation of more crystals which fall deeper into the dentinal tubule. These crystals form a barrier and slow the advancement of caries. After these protective responses, the dentin is considered sclerotic.

Fluids within dentinal tubules are believed to be the mechanism by which pain receptors are triggered within the pulp of the tooth. Since sclerotic dentin prevents the passage of such fluids, pain that would otherwise serve as a warning of the invading bacteria may not develop at first. Consequently, dental caries may progress for a long period of time without any sensitivity of the tooth, allowing for greater loss of tooth structure.

Tertiary Dentin: In response to dental caries, there may be production of more dentin toward the direction of the pulp. This new dentin is referred to as tertiary dentin. Tertiary dentin is produced to protect the pulp for as long as possible from the advancing bacteria. As more tertiary dentin is produced, the size of the pulp decreases. This type of dentin has been subdivided according to the presence or absence of the original odontoblasts. If the odontoblasts survive long enough to react to the dental caries, then the dentin produced is called "reactionary" dentin. If the odontoblasts are killed, the dentin produced is called "reparative" dentin. In the case of reparative dentin, other cells are needed to assume the role of the destroyed odontoblasts. Growth factors, especially TGF-â, are thought to initiate the production of reparative dentin by fibroblasts and mesenchymal cells of the pulp. Reparative dentin is produced at an average of 1.5 ìm/day, but can be increased to 3.5 ìm/day.

The resulting dentin contains irregularly shaped dentinal tubules which may not line up with existing dentinal tubules. This diminishes the ability for dental caries to progress within the dentinal tubules.

Pneumonia

Pneumonia is an inflammatory condition of the lung. It is often characterized as including inflammation of the parenchyma of the lung (that is, the alveoli) and abnormal alveolar filling with fluid (consolidation and exudation).

The alveoli are microscopic air filled sacs in the lungs responsible for gas exchange. Pneumonia can result from a variety of causes, including infection with bacteria, viruses, fungi, or parasites, and chemical or physical injury to the lungs. Its cause may also be officially described as unknown when infectious causes have been excluded.

Typical symptoms associated with pneumonia include cough, chest pain, fever, and difficulty in breathing. Diagnostic tools include x-rays and examination of the sputum. Treatment depends on the cause of pneumonia; bacterial pneumonia is treated with antibiotics. Pneumonia is common, occurring in all age groups, and is a leading cause of death among the young, the old, and the chronically ill. Vaccines to prevent certain types of pneumonia are available. The prognosis depends on the type of pneumonia, the treatment, any complications, and the person's underlying health.

Classification

Pneumonias can be classified in several ways. The primary system of classification is the combined clinical classification, which combines factors such as age, risk factors for certain microorganisms, the presence of underlying lung disease or systemic disease, and whether the person has recently been hospitalized. Other classifications include according to the anatomic changes that can be found in the lungs during autopsies, based on the microbial cause, and a radiological classification.

Clinical

Traditionally, clinicians have classified pneumonia by clinical characteristics, dividing them into "acute" (less than three weeks duration) and "chronic" pneumonias. This is useful because chronic pneumonias tend to be either non-infectious, or mycobacterial, fungal, or mixed bacterial infections caused by airway obstruction. Acute pneumonias are further divided into the classic bacterial bronchopneumonias (such as *Streptococcus pneumoniae*), the atypical pneumonias (such as the interstitial pneumonitis of *Mycoplasma pneumoniae* or *Chlamydia pneumoniae*), and the aspiration pneumonia syndromes. Chronic pneumonias, on the other hand, mainly include those of *Nocardia*, *Actinomyces* and *Blastomyces dermatitidis*, as well as the granulomatous pneumonias (*Mycobacterium tuberculosis* and atypical mycobacteria, *Histoplasma capsulatum* and *Coccidioides immitis*).

The combined clinical classification, now the most commonly used classification scheme, attempts to identify a person's risk factors when he or she first comes to medical attention. The advantage of this classification scheme over previous systems is that it can help guide the selection of appropriate initial treatments even before the microbiologic cause of the pneumonia is known. There are two broad categories of pneumonia in this scheme: community-acquired pneumonia and hospital-acquired pneumonia. A recently introduced type of healthcare-associated pneumonia (in patients living outside the hospital who have recently been in close contact with the health care system) lies between these two categories.

Community-acquired

Community-acquired pneumonia (CAP) is infectious pneumonia in a person who has not recently been hospitalized. CAP is the most common type of pneumonia. The most common causes of CAP vary depending on a person's age, but they include *Streptococcus pneumoniae*, viruses, the atypical bacteria, and *Haemophilus influenzae*. Overall, *Streptococcus pneumoniae* is the most common cause of community-acquired pneumonia worldwide. Gram-negative bacteria cause CAP in certain at-risk populations. CAP is the fourth most common cause of death in the United Kingdom and the sixth in the United States. The term "walking pneumonia" has been used to describe a type of community-acquired pneumonia of less severity (because the sufferer can continue to "walk" rather than require hospitalization). Walking pneumonia is usually caused by the atypical bacterium, *Mycoplasma pneumoniae*.

Hospital-acquired

Hospital-acquired pneumonia, also called nosocomial pneumonia, is pneumonia acquired during or after hospitalization for another illness or procedure with onset at least 72 hrs after admission. The causes, microbiology, treatment and prognosis are different from those of community-acquired pneumonia. Up to 5% of patients admitted to a hospital for other causes subsequently develop pneumonia. Hospitalized patients may have many risk factors for pneumonia, including mechanical ventilation, prolonged malnutrition, underlying heart and lung diseases, decreased amounts of stomach acid, and immune disturbances. Additionally, the microorganisms a person is exposed to in a hospital are often different from those at home. Hospital-acquired microorganisms may include resistant bacteria such as MRSA, *Pseudomonas*, *Enterobacter*, and *Serratia*. Because individuals with hospital-acquired pneumonia usually have underlying illnesses and are exposed to more dangerous bacteria, it tends to be more deadly than community-acquired pneumonia. Ventilator-associated pneumonia (VAP) is a subset of hospital-acquired pneumonia. VAP is pneumonia which occurs after at least 48 hours of intubation and mechanical ventilation.

Other Types

- Bronchiolitis obliterans organizing pneumonia (BOOP)

  BOOP is caused by inflammation of the small airways of the lungs. It is also known as cryptogenic organizing pneumonitis (COP).

- Eosinophilic pneumonia

  Eosinophilic pneumonia is invasion of the lung by eosinophils, a particular kind of white blood cell. Eosinophilic pneumonia often occurs in response to infection with a parasite or after exposure to certain types of environmental factors.

- Chemical pneumonia

  Chemical pneumonia (usually called chemical pneumonitis) is caused by chemical toxicants such as pesticides, which may enter the body by inhalation or by skin contact. When the toxic substance is an oil, the pneumonia may be called *lipoid pneumonia.*

- Aspiration pneumonia

  Aspiration pneumonia (or aspiration pneumonitis) is caused by aspirating foreign objects which are usually oral or gastric contents, either while eating, or after reflux or vomiting which results in bronchopneumonia. The resulting lung inflammation is not an infection but can contribute to one, since the material aspirated may contain anaerobic bacteria or other unusual causes of pneumonia.

Aspiration is a leading cause of death among hospital and nursing home patients, since they often cannot adequately protect their airways and may have otherwise impaired defenses.

- Dust pneumonia

  Dust pneumonia describes disorders caused by excessive exposure to dust storms, particularly during the Dust Bowl in the United States. With dust pneumonia, dust settles all the way into the alveoli of the lungs, stopping the cilia from moving and preventing the lungs from ever clearing themselves.
- Necrotizing pneumonia, although overlapping with many other classifications, includes pneumonias that cause substantial necrosis of lung cells, and sometimes even lung abscess. Implicated bacteria are extremely commonly anaerobic bacteria, with or without additional facultatively anaerobic ones like Staphylococcus aureus, Klebsiella pneumoniae and Streptococcus pyogenes. Type 3 pneumococcus is uncommonly implicated.
- Opportunistic pneumonia includes those that frequently strike immunocompromised victims. Main pathogens are cytomegalovirus, Pneumocystis jiroveci, Mycobacterium avium-intracellulare, invasive aspergillosis, invasive candidiasis, as well as the "usual bacteria" that strike immunocompetent people as well.
- Double pneumonia is a historical term for acute lung injury (ALI) or acute respiratory distress syndrome (ARDS). However, the term was, and is used still, especially by lay people, to denote pneumonia affecting both lungs. Accordingly, the term 'double pneumonia' is more likely to be used to describe bilateral pneumonia than it is ALI or ARDS.
- Severe acute respiratory syndrome (SARS): is a highly contagious and deadly type of pneumonia which first occurred in 2002 after initial outbreaks in China. SARS is caused by the SARS coronavirus, a previously unknown pathogen. Last recorded occurrence was in 2003.

Other

Initial descriptions of pneumonia focused on the anatomic or pathologic appearance of the lung, either by direct inspection at autopsy or by its appearance under a microscope.

- A *lobar* pneumonia is an infection that only involves a single lobe, or section, of a lung. Lobar pneumonia is often due to *Streptococcus pneumoniae* (though *Klebsiella pneumoniae* is also possible.)
- *Multilobar* pneumonia involves more than one lobe, and it often causes a more severe illness.
- Bronchial pneumonia affects the lungs in patches around the tubes (bronchi or bronchioles).
- *Interstitial* pneumonia involves the areas in between the alveoli, and it may be called "interstitial pneumonitis." It is more likely to be caused by viruses or by atypical bacteria.

The discovery of x-rays made it possible to determine the anatomic type of pneumonia without direct examination of the lungs at autopsy and led to the development of a radiological classification. Early investigators distinguished between typical lobar pneumonia and atypical (e.g. Chlamydophila) or viral pneumonia using the location, distribution, and appearance of the opacities they saw on chest x-rays. Certain x-ray findings can be used to help predict the course of illness, although it is not possible to clearly determine the microbiologic cause of a pneumonia with x-rays alone. With the advent of modern microbiology, classification based upon the causative microorganism became possible. Determining which microorganism is causing an individual's pneumonia is an important step in deciding treatment type and length. Sputum cultures, blood cultures, tests on respiratory secretions, and specific blood tests are used to determine the microbiologic classification. Because such laboratory testing typically takes several days, microbiologic classification is usually not possible at the time of initial diagnosis.

Chapter

6

Microbiology Applied in Food

Quality Assurance and Sanitation Programs in Food Industry

Since the late 1970s, the food industry has emphasized an organized sanitation program that monitors the microbiology of raw ingredients in production plants and the wholesomeness and safety of the finished products, in an effort to maintain or upgrade the acceptability of its food products.

As consumers become better informed and more sophisticated, it is even more vital for the food industry to develop an effective quality assurance (QA) and sanitation program. The efforts of regulatory agencies in the field of sanitation and food microbiology have been responsible for the food industry's implementation of voluntary quality assurance programs. Food scientists have also had a positive impact on quality assurance programs because many of these professionals have joined various companies in the food industry. Their efforts have been instrumental in the adoption and/or upgrading of quality assurance programs for the organizations they represent.

In its initial stages, quality assurance was primarily a quality control function, acting as an arm of manufacturing. It has now evolved to formidable force within executive structure of large food firms and has emerged into broad spectrum of activities. A quality assurance program provides the avenue to establish checks and balances in the areas of food safety, public health, technical expertise, and legal matters affecting food manufacturing firms. Activities related to food sanitation include sanitation inspections, products releases and holds, packaging sanitation, and product recalls and withdrawals.

A quality assurance program that emphasizes sanitation is vital to the growth of a food establishment. If foods are to compete effectively in the market place, established hygienic standards must be strictly maintained. However, it is sometimes impractical for production personnel to measure and monitor sanitation while maintaining a high level of productivity and efficiency. Thus, an effective quality assurance program should be available to monitor, within established priorities, each phase of the operation. All personnel should incorporate the team concept to attain established sanitary standard, ensuring that food products in the market place are safe.

Food Safety – SSOP (Standard Sanitation Operating Procedures)

Without a properly designed system to maintain sanitation, all other systems, including HACCP, will fail. It is this reason that all working meat establishments must have an active and approved SSOP program that has been signed and dated.

The SSOP consists of step-by-step procedures explaining exactly how sanitation will be maintained within the food establishment. The SSOP basically works as a plan for preventing contamination of product – derived from equipment or employee's product handling practices. The main objective of the SSOP is to allow a wholesome, safe product to be produced within a sanitary environment.

SSOP Planning and Design

The most important components of a properly developed SSOP are the Design and Execution. Each SSOP is "plant specific," meaning it was designed for a specific establishment. It is possible to modify a SSOP that has already been designed, or one can be created specifically in style of the establishment in which it will be used. As long as it meets regulatory requirements, is approved, and has been proven to be a working plan, it should be acceptable.

When deciding on the SSOP design, a general idea of the design and operations of the establishment must be known. For example, one would want to focus more on sanitation in a room that packs fully cooked product (such as bologna or sandwich meat) than that of a storage room. The storage room must be monitored, but probably not as much as the room that packs fully cooked product. Other equipment such as saws, grinders, table tops, cubing machines, knifes, and sterilizers, are examples of equipment that would need to be included in the first step of the SSOP design. There must be cleaning steps identifying how these food-contact utensils are cleaned and sanitized.

The SSOP Outline

The written SSOP should begin with a description of the establishments SSOP program. This description should give a clear and brief understanding of the establishments standard sanitation operating procedures, including: the establishment name, city and state in which the establishment is located, an approximate number of employees working within the establishment, any special safeguards (such as good manufacturing practices and pest control programs), management structures, equipment and facilities, and a recordkeeping system.

The next step will be to describe the pre-operational sanitation check (before operations begin) where designated employees will actually perform a visual check and cleaning techniques of the equipment and facilities – placing primary focus on food-contact surfaces, and the operational sanitation check (after operations begin) where sanitation is monitored and documented during processing hours. The SSOP "checks" are normally performed at least twice a day. These checks include a "pre-operational sanitation check" (performed before operations begin) and an "operational check" (performed during operations). Each sanitation check is performed by the designated employee and their findings are documented within a SSOP recordkeeping system. It is this recordkeeping system, as well as the actual monitoring of the SSOP, that is reviewed by USDA Inspection Personnel to verify the establishment is providing a clean and sanitary environment to produce their product.

The Pre-Operational Sanitation Check (Pre-Op)

The pre-operational sanitation check (also known as the "pre-op") is performed prior to operations. Before any food product enters a room, the pre-op should be performed in that room to verify that facilities, equipment, and utensils were properly cleaned after the previous work day. As mentioned above, all equipment and utensils are cleaned and sanitized before operations begin.

The pre-op often consists of a general walk-through of the establishment to verify the facilities, all equipment, utensils, and all food contact surfaces that may come in direct or indirect contact with the product are clean and acceptable. Often, plant personnel will use a pump sprayer, equipped with an approved sanitizer to spray all equipment and utensils before operations begin. This will likely eliminate most of any bacterial growth that may have occurred between the clean-up and the pre-op.

The Operational Sanitation Check

The operational sanitation check is performed similar to the pre-operational sanitation check, but it is performed during operations (while product is being processed), and at least once per day. The primary objective of the operational sanitation check is to verify that processing is being performed under sanitary conditions (including employee handling) to prevent any direct or cross-contamination of food products. This includes food contact surfaces as well as non-food contact surfaces. As with the pre-operational sanitation check, the results or findings of the operational sanitation check must be documented on some form of SSOP report.

SSOP Forms and Recordkeeping

It is entirely up to the establishment as to how their SSOP forms and record keeping systems are designed. The forms will be acceptable as long as they show documentation of all findings (or no findings), and any corrective actions that were needed upon a noted deficiency within the SSOP. There are no specific standards as to how the forms are designed.

Final Thoughts – Standard Sanitation Operating Procedures

Perform the sanitation checks exactly as described in the approved SSOP. Properly and accurately record any findings (or no findings if none) and complete and properly file the form(s) at the proper times. While SSOP Checks are being performed, it is recommended to use a flashlight and have the proper form(s) ready so they can be completed at the proper times. Double check the "hard-to-get" places for meat and fat debris – if these are overlooked the meat inspector will likely find them!

Identify and record any corrective actions as listed in the plant SSOP for any non-food contact surface deficiencies. Inspection Personnel will gladly assist in answering any questions that may arise pertaining to the SSOP. If there is anything that is not understood, ask the USDA Inspector. They will assist through outreach.

Food-borne Microbes and Food Poisoning

Bacteria

Of all the microorganisms, bacteria are the greatest threat to food safety. Bacteria are single-celled, living organisms that can grow quickly at favourable temperatures. However, some bacteria are useful e.g. these that to make foods like cheese, buttermilk, sauerkraut, pickles, and yogurt. Other bacteria are infectious disease-causing agents called pathogens, that use the nutrients found in potentially hazardous foods to multiply.

Some bacteria are not infectious on their own, but when they multiply in potentially hazardous food, they eject toxins that poison humans when the food is eaten. Food handling practices are risky when they allow harmful bacteria to contaminate and grow in food. If you touch a potentially hazardous food during preparation, you may transfer several thousand bacteria to its surface.

Under the right conditions, bacteria can double every 10 to 30 minutes. A single bacterium will double with each division—two become four, four become eight, and so on. A single cell can become billions in 10 to 12 hours.

Salmonella

Foods Associated with Salmonella: Raw poultry products, eggs, pork, processed meats. Less commonly, Salmonella has been found to be associated with raw fruits and vegetables.

Cause of illness: Infection with Salmonella species.

Incubation period: 12-24 hours.

Characteristics of Illness: Fever, cramps, diarrhea and sometimes vomiting.

Possible contaminant: Meat, poultry, egg or milk products.

Onset: Illness may begin between 7 hrs to 3 days after eating contaminated food.

Duration: Illness may last 2-3 days.;

Prevention of Illness:

- Avoid cross-contamination of ready-to-eat foods with raw meats or their juices.
- Thoroughly cook meat and poultry.
- Cook eggs thoroughly and never eat runny yolks or raw eggs.

- Always refrigerate processed meat products.
- Wash fruits and vegetables thoroughly.

Campylobacter

Foods Associated with Campylobacter: Raw chicken and raw milk.

Cause of illness: Infection, even with low numbers.

Incubation period: One to seven days.

Characteristics of Illness: Diarrhea, often associated with fever, abdominal pain, nausea, headache and muscle pain. Illness can appear very similar to Salmonellosis.

Possible contaminant: Raw milk, eggs, poultry, raw beef, cake icing, water

Onset: Illness may begin between 2-5 days after eating contaminated food.

Duration: Illness may last 7-10 days.

Staphylococcus Aureus

Foods Associated with Staphylococcus aureus: This bacteria has been associated with a wide range of foods, including meat and meat products, poultry and egg products, salads such as egg, tuna, potato and macaroni, cream-filled bakery products and pies, sandwich fillings and milk and dairy products. In general, Staph poisoning often occurs when a food has been handled a great deal (such as the chopping and handling involved in making a salad or sandwich) and is then left at temperatures above refrigeration which allow the bacteria to multiply and produce toxin.

Cause of illness: Toxin produced by certain strains of Staphylococcus aureus:

Incubation period: One-six hours.

Characteristics of Illness: Vomiting, diarrhea and abdominal cramps.

Onset: Illness may begin within 3-8 hrs. after eating contaminated food.

Duration: Illness usually lasts about 2 days.

Prevention of Illness:

- Always wash hands well when preparing foods.
- Keep foods refrigerated.

Listeria Monocytogenes

Foods Associated with Listeria monocytogenes: Raw milk, raw meats and raw vegetables. Ice cream, soft-ripened cheeses, smoked fish, lunch meats, hot dogs and refrigerated salad-type products. This organism is unique in that it is able to grow even at refrigerated temperatures and so, while refrigeration of foods will slow the growth of Listeria, it will not stop it completely.

Cause of illness: Infection with Listeria monocytogenes.

Characteristics of Illness: In healthy individuals this organism may result in diarrhea, vomiting and nausea. However, in immunocompromised individuals (the very young, the elderly, pregnant women, those with AIDS or undergoing cancer treatment) Listeriosis may first appear as mild flu-like symptoms, but may then be followed by septicemia, meningitis, encephalitis and spontaneous abortion or stillbirth in pregnant women.

Possible contaminant: Vegetables, milk, cheese, meat, seafood.

Onset: Illness may occur anywhere from 12 hrs to a few weeks after contaminated food is consumed.

Duration: In otherwise healthy individuals, mild symptoms may disappear in a day or two, but medical attention is required for immunosuppressed individuals who develop the above mentioned complications.

Prevention of Illness:

- Wash fresh fruits and vegetables thoroughly under running water.
- Keep foods refrigerated to slow the growth of Listeria, if it is present.
- Immunocompromised individuals should try to avoid eating implicated foods, such as soft-ripened cheeses or lunchmeat products.
- Pasteurize milk, cook foods properly, avoid cross- contamination; use sanitary practices.

E. Coli 0157:H7

Foods Associated with E. coli O157:H7: Undercooked raw meat, apple cider, raw milk and raw produce.

Cause of illness: Strain of enteropathic E. coli.

Incubation period: Two to four days.

Characteristics of Illness: Severe cramping and diarrhea which is initially watery but becomes grossly bloody.

Possible contaminant: Ground beef, raw milk, alfalfa sprouts, unpasteurized fruit juices, dry-cured salami, lettuce, meat, and cheese curds.

Onset: Illness may occur anywhere between 1 to 10 days after eating contaminated food, but usually occurs between 3 to 4 days.

Prevention of Illness:

- Cook ground meat thoroughly such that the to an internal reaches minimum temp of 75°C.
- Wash fresh fruits and vegetables thoroughly with running water.
- Do not drink unpasteurized milk.
- Do not drink unpasteurized apple cider unless it is well refrigerated.

Clostridium Botulinum

Foods Associated with Clostridium botulinum: Improperly processed home canned foods. and Low-acid canned foods, meats, sausage, fish.

Cause of illness: Toxin produced by Clostridium botulinum.

Incubation period: 12 to 36 hours.

Characteristics of Illness: Symptoms include double vision, vertigo, inability to swallow, Nausea, vomiting, diarrhea, fatigue, headache, dry mouth, speech difficulty and progressive respiratory paralysis or respiratory failure. Nausea may also be present initially.

Onset: Symptoms may begin within 18 hrs to 2 days of ingesting the toxin.

Duration: Greater than 65% of cases are fatal. In non-fatal botulism poisoning, recovery may take weeks to years, depending upon the severity of the poisoning.

Clostridium Perfringens

Foods Associated with Clostridium perfringens: Meat and/ or gravy dishes are most often associated with this type of food borne illness. Generally C. perfringens poisoning occurs when such meat dishes are not cooked to high enough temperatures and then are allowed to sit out at room temperature for serving for an extended period of time.

Cause of illness: Contamination of drinking water or milk.

Incubation period:8 to 24 hours.

Characteristics of Illness: Abdominal cramping and diarrhea, headache, chills.

Possible contaminant: Meat, poultry, and other foods held for serving at warm, but not hot, temperatures

Onset: Illness may begin between 8 to 22 hrs after ingesting contaminated food.

Duration: Illness may last 1-2 days.

Bacillus Cereus

Foods Associated with Bacillus cereus: Rice and grain products, dairy products such as milk, cream, custards and dried milk.

Characteristics of Illness: Bacillus cereus may cause two different types of illness. The first is know as the Diarrheal illness, which results in diarrhea and abdominal cramps occurring within 6 to 15 hrs of eating contaminated food. This illness may persist up to about 24 hours and resembles Clostridium perfringens food poisoning. The second type of illness caused by Bacillus cereus is know as the Emetic illness and results in nausea and vomiting within 3-6 hours of eating contaminated food. This illness also lasts about 24 hrs and it tends to resemble Staphylococcal food poisoning.

There are two types of food poisoning: infectious agent and toxic agent. Food infection refers to the presence of bacteria or other microbes which infect the body after consumption. Food intoxication refers to the ingestion of toxins contained within the food, including bacterially produced exotoxins, which can happen even when the microbe that produced the toxin is no longer present or able to cause infection. In spite of the common term food poisoning, most cases are caused by a variety of pathogenic bacteria, viruses, or parasites that contaminate food, rather than chemical or natural toxins.

Foodborne illness usually arises from improper handling, preparation, or food storage. Good hygiene practices before, during, and after food preparation can reduce the chances of contracting an illness. There is a general consensus in the public health community that regular hand-washing is one of the most effective defences against the spread of foodborne illness. The action of monitoring food to ensure that it will not cause foodborne illness is known as food safety. Foodborne disease can also be caused by a large variety of toxins that affect the environment. For foodborne illness caused by chemicals. Foodborne illness can also be caused by pesticides or medicines in food and naturally toxic substances like poisonous mushrooms or reef fish.

Bacteria

Bacteria are a common cause of foodborne illness. In the United Kingdom during 2000 the individual bacteria involved were as follows: *Campylobacter jejuni* 77.3%, *Salmonella* 20.9%, *Escherichia coli O157:H7* 1.4%, and all others less than 0.1%.

In the past, bacterial infections were thought to be more prevalent because few places had the capability to test for norovirus and no active surveillance was being done for this particular agent. Symptoms for bacterial infections are delayed because the bacteria need time to multiply. They are usually not seen until 12–72 hours or more after eating contaminated food.

Most common bacterial foodborne pathogens are:

- *Campylobacter jejuni* which can lead to secondary Guillain–Barre syndrome and periodontitis
- *Clostridium perfringens*, the "cafeteria germ"
- *Salmonella* spp. – its *S. typhimurium* infection is caused by consumption of eggs or poultry that are not adequately cooked or by other interactive human-animal pathogens
- *Escherichia coli O157:H7* enterohemorrhagic (EHEC) which causes hemolytic-uremic syndrome.

Other common bacterial foodborne pathogens are:

- *Bacillus cereus*
- *Escherichia coli*, other virulence properties, such as enteroinvasive (EIEC), enteropathogenic (EPEC), enterotoxigenic (ETEC), enteroaggregative (EAEC or EAgEC)
- *Listeria monocytogenes*
- *Shigella* spp.
- *Staphylococcus aureus*
- *Streptococcus*
- *Vibrio cholerae*, including O1 and non-O1
- *Vibrio parahaemolyticus*
- *Vibrio vulnificus*
- *Yersinia enterocolitica* and *Yersinia pseudotuberculosis*.

Less common bacterial agents:

- *Brucella* spp.
- *Corynebacterium ulcerans*
- *Coxiella burnetii* or Q fever
- *Plesiomonas shigelloides.*

Exotoxins

In addition to disease caused by direct bacterial infection, some foodborne illnesses are caused by exotoxins which are excreted by the cell as the bacterium grows. Exotoxins can produce illness even when the microbes that produced them have been killed. Symptoms typically appear after 1–6 hours depending on the amount of toxin ingested.

- *Clostridium botulinum*
- *Clostridium perfringens*
- *Staphylococcus aureus*
- *Bacillus cereus.*

For example *Staphylococcus aureus* produces a toxin that causes intense vomiting. The rare but potentially deadly disease botulism occurs when the anaerobic bacterium *Clostridium botulinum* grows in improperly canned low-acid foods and produces botulin, a powerful paralytic toxin.

Pseudoalteromonas tetraodonis, certain species of Pseudomonas and Vibrio, and some other bacteria, produce the lethal tetrodotoxin, which is present in the tissues of some living animal species rather than being a product of decomposition.

Mycotoxins and Alimentary Mycotoxicoses

The term alimentary mycotoxicoses refers to the effect of poisoning by Mycotoxins through food consumption. Mycotoxins sometimes have important effects on human and animal health. For example, an outbreak which occurred in the UK in 1960 caused the death of 100,000 turkeys which had consumed aflatoxin-contaminated peanut meal. In the USSR in World War II, 5000 people died due to Alimentary Toxic Aleukia (ALA). The common foodborne Mycotoxins include:

- Aflatoxins – originated from Aspergillus parasiticus and Aspergillus flavus. They are frequently found in tree nuts, peanuts, maize, sorghum and other oilseeds, including corn and cottonseeds. The pronounced forms of Aflatoxins are those of B1, B2, G1, and G2, amongst which Aflatoxin B1 predominantly targets the liver, which will result in necrosis, cirrhosis, and carcinoma. In the US, the acceptable level of total aflatoxins in foods is less than 20 μg/kg, except for Aflatoxin M1 in milk, which should be less than 0.5 μg/kg. The official document can be found at FDA's website.

- Altertoxins – are those of Alternariol (AOH), Alternariol methyl ether (AME), Altenuene (ALT), Altertoxin-1 (ATX-1), Tenuazonic acid (TeA) and Radicinin (RAD), originated from Alternaria spp. Some of the toxins can be present in sorghum, ragi, wheat and tomatoes. Some research has shown that the toxins can be easily cross-contaminated between grain commodities, suggesting that manufacturing and storage of grain commodities is a critical practice.
- Citrinin
- Citreoviridin
- Cyclopiazonic acid
- Cytochalasins
- Ergot alkaloids/Ergopeptine alkaloids – Ergotamine
- Fumonisins – Crop corn can be easily contaminated by the fungi Fusarium moniliforme, and its Fumonisin B1 will cause Leukoencephalomalacia (LEM) in horses, Pulmonary edema syndrome (PES) in pigs, liver cancer in rats and Esophageal cancer in humans. For human and animal health, both the FDA and the EC have regulated the content levels of toxins in food and animal feed.
- Fusaric acid
- Fusarochromanone
- Kojic acid
- Lolitrem alkaloids
- Moniliformin
- 3-Nitropropionic acid
- Nivalenol
- Ochratoxins – In Australia, The Limit of Reporting (LOR) level for Ochratoxin A (OTA) analyses in 20th Australian Total Diet Survey was 1 μg/kg, whereas the EC restricts the content of OTA to 5 μg/kg in cereal commodities, 3 μg/kg in processed products and 10 μg/kg in dried vine fruits.
- Oosporeine

- Patulin – Currently, this toxin has been advisably regulated on fruit products. The EC and the FDA have limited it to under 50 μg/kg for fruit juice and fruit nectar, while limits of 25 μg/kg for solid-contained fruit products and 10 μg/kg for baby foods were specified by the EC.
- Phomopsins
- Sporidesmin A
- Sterigmatocystin
- Tremorgenic mycotoxins – Five of them have been reported to be associated with molds found in fermented meats. These are Fumitremorgen B, Paxilline, Penitrem A, Verrucosidin, and Verruculogen.
- Trichothecenes – sourced from Cephalosporium, Fusarium, Myrothecium, Stachybotrys and Trichoderma. The toxins are usually found in molded maize, wheat, corn, peanuts and rice, or animal feed of hay and straw. Four trichothecenes, T-2 toxin, HT-2 toxin, diacetoxyscirpenol (DAS) and deoxynivalenol (DON) have been most commonly encountered by humans and animals. The consequences of oral intake of, or dermal exposure to, the toxins will result in Alimentary toxic aleukia, neutropenia, aplastic anemia, thrombocytopenia and/or skin irritation. In 1993, the FDA issued a document for the content limits of DON in food and animal feed at an advisory level. In 2003, US published a patent that is very promising for farmers to produce a trichothecene-resistant crop.
- Zearalenone
- Zearalenols.

Emerging Foodborne Pathogens

Many foodborne illnesses remain poorly understood. Approximately sixty percent of outbreaks are caused by unknown sources.

- *Aeromonas hydrophila*, *Aeromonas caviae*, *Aeromonas sobria*.

Preventing Bacterial Food Poisoning

Prevention is mainly the role of the state, through the definition of strict rules of hygiene and a public services of veterinary surveying of animal products in the food chain, from farming to the transformation industry and delivery (shops and restaurants). This regulation includes:

- traceability: in a final product, it must be possible to know the origin of the ingredients (originating farm, identification of the harvesting or of the animal) and where and when it was processed; the origin of the illness can thus be tracked and solved (and possibly penalized), and the final products can be removed from the sale if a problem is detected;
- enforcement of hygiene procedures like HACCP and the "cold chain";
- power of control and of law enforcement of veterinarians.

In August 2006, the United States Food and Drug Administration approved Phage therapy which involves spraying meat with viruses that infect bacteria, and thus preventing infection. This has raised concerns, because without mandatory labelling consumers wouldn't be aware that meat and poultry products have been treated with the spray. At home, prevention mainly consists of good food safety practices. Many forms of bacterial poisoning can be prevented even if food is contaminated by cooking it sufficiently, and either eating it quickly or refrigerating it effectively. Many toxins, however, are not destroyed by heat treatment.

Viruses

Viral infections make up perhaps one third of cases of food poisoning in developed countries. In the US, more than 50% of cases are viral and noroviruses are the most common foodborne illness, causing 57% of outbreaks in 2004. Foodborne viral infection are usually of intermediate (1–3 days) incubation period, causing illnesses which are self-limited in otherwise healthy individuals, and are similar to the bacterial forms described above.

- Enterovirus
- Hepatitis A is distinguished from other viral causes by its prolonged (2–6 week) incubation period and its ability to spread beyond the stomach and intestines, into the liver. It often induces jaundice, or yellowing of the skin, and rarely leads to chronic liver dysfunction. The virus has been found to cause the infection due to the consumption of fresh-cut produce which has fecal contamination.
- Hepatitis E
- Norovirus
- Rotavirus.

Parasites

Most foodborne parasites are zoonoses.

- Platyhelminthes:
  - *Diphyllobothrium* sp.
  - *Nanophyetus* sp.
  - *Taenia saginata*
  - *Taenia solium*
  - *Fasciola hepatica.*
- Nematode:
  - *Anisakis* sp.
  - *Ascaris lumbricoides*
  - *Eustrongylides* sp.
  - *Trichinella spiralis*
  - *Trichuris trichiura.*
- Protozoa:
  - *Acanthamoeba* and other free-living amoebae
  - *Cryptosporidium parvum*
  - *Cyclospora cayetanensis*
  - *Entamoeba histolytica*
  - *Giardia lamblia*
  - *Sarcocystis hominis*
  - *Sarcocystis suihominis*
  - *Toxoplasma gondii.*

Natural Toxins

Several foods can naturally contain toxins, many of which are not produced by bacteria. Plants in particular may be toxic; animals which are naturally poisonous to eat are rare. In evolutionary terms, animals can escape being eaten by fleeing; plants can use only passive defences such as poisons and distasteful substances, for example capsaicin in chili peppers and pungent sulfur compounds in garlic and onions. Most animal poisons are not synthesised by the animal, but acquired by eating poisonous plants to which the animal is immune, or by bacterial action.

- Alkaloids
- Ciguatera poisoning

- Grayanotoxin (honey intoxication)
- Mushroom toxins
- Phytohaemagglutinin (red kidney bean poisoning; destroyed by boiling)
- Pyrrolizidine alkaloids
- Shellfish toxin, including paralytic shellfish poisoning, diarrhetic shellfish poisoning, neurotoxic shellfish poisoning, amnesic shellfish poisoning and ciguatera fish poisoning
- Scombrotoxin
- Tetrodotoxin (fugu fish poisoning).

Some plants contain substances which are toxic in large doses, but have therapeutic properties in appropriate dosages.

- Foxglove contains cardiac glycosides.
- Poisonous hemlock (conium) has medicinal uses.

Other Pathogenic Agents

- Prions, resulting in Creutzfeldt-Jakob disease.

"Ptomaine Poisoning"

An early theory on the causes of food poisoning involved *ptomaines* (from Greek *ptôma*, "fall, fallen body, corpse"), alkaloids found in decaying animal and vegetable matter. While some alkaloids do cause poisoning, the discovery of bacteria left the ptomaine theory obsolete and the word *ptomaine* is no longer used scientifically.

Mechanism

Incubation Period

The delay between consumption of a contaminated food and appearance of the first symptoms of illness is called the incubation period. This ranges from hours to days (and rarely months or even years, such as in the case of Listeriosis or Creutzfeldt-Jacob disease), depending on the agent, and on how much was consumed. If symptoms occur within 1–6 hours after eating the food, it suggests that it is caused by a bacterial toxin or a chemical rather than live bacteria.

The long incubation period of many foodborne illnesses tends to cause sufferers to attribute their symptoms to "stomach flu".

During the incubation period, microbes pass through the stomach into the intestine, attach to the cells lining the intestinal walls, and begin to multiply there. Some types of microbes stay in the intestine, some produce a toxin that is absorbed into the bloodstream, and some can directly invade the deeper body tissues. The symptoms produced depend on the type of microbe.

Infectious Dose

The infectious dose is the amount of agent that must be consumed to give rise to symptoms of foodborne illness, and varies according to the agent and the consumer's age and overall health. In the case of *Salmonella* a relatively large inoculum of 1 million to 1 billion organisms is necessary to produce symptoms in healthy human volunteers, as *Salmonellae* are very sensitive to acid. An unusually high stomach pH level (low acidity) greatly reduces the number of bacteria required to cause symptoms by a factor of between 10 and 100.

Epidemiology

Every year there are an estimated 76 million foodborne illnesses in the United States (26,000 cases for 100,000 inhabitants), 2 million in the United Kingdom (3,400 cases for 100,000 inhabitants) and 750,000 in France (1,220 cases for 100,000 inhabitants).

United States

In the United States, using FoodNet data from 1996–1998, the CDCP estimated there were 76 million foodborne illnesses (26,000 cases for 100,000 inhabitants):

- 325,000 were hospitalized (111 per 100,000 inhabitants);
- 5,000 people died (1.7 per 100,000 inhabitants.).
- Major pathogens from foodborne illness in the United States cost upwards of US $35 billion in medical costs and lost productivity (1997).

France

In France, for 750,000 cases(1,210 per 100,000 inhabitants):

- 70,000 people consulted in the emergency department of an hospital (113 per 100,000 inhabitants.);
- 113,000 people were hospitalized (24 per 100,000 inhabitants);
- 400 people died (0.9 per 100,000 inhabitants).

Australia

In Australia, there are an estimated 5.4 million cases of food-borne illness every year, causing:

- 18,000 hospitalizations
- 120 deaths
- 2.1 million lost days off work
- 1.2 million doctor consultations
- 300,000 prescriptions for antibiotics.

Outbreaks

The vast majority of reported cases of foodborne illness occur as individual or sporadic cases. The origin of most sporadic cases is undetermined. In the United States, where people eat outside the home frequently, most outbreaks (58%) originate from commercial food facilities (2004 FoodNet data). An outbreak is defined as occurring when two or more people experience similar illness after consuming food from a common source.

Often, a combination of events contributes to an outbreak, for example, food might be left at room temperature for many hours, allowing bacteria to multiply which is compounded by inadequate cooking which results in a failure to kill the dangerously elevated bacterial levels.

Outbreaks are usually identified when those affected know each other. However, more and more, outbreaks are identified by public health staff from unexpected increases in laboratory results for certain strains of bacteria. Outbreak detection and investigation in the United States is primarily handled by local health jurisdictions and is inconsistent from district to district. It is estimated that 1–2% of outbreaks are detected.

Pathogens and Antibiotics

A pathogen an infectious agent, or more commonly germ, is a biological agent that causes disease to its host. There are several substrates including *pathways* whereby pathogens can invade a host; the principal pathways have different episodic time frames, but soil contamination has the longest or most persistent potential for harboring a pathogen.

The body contains many natural orders of defence against some of the common pathogens (such as *Pneumocystis*) in the form of the human immune system and by some "helpful" bacteria present in the human body's normal flora. However, if the immune system or "good" bacteria is damaged in any way (such as by chemotherapy, human immunodeficiency virus (HIV), or antibiotics being taken to kill other pathogens), pathogenic bacteria that were being held at bay can proliferate and cause harm to the host. Such cases are called opportunistic infection.

Some pathogens (such as the bacterium *Yersinia pestis* which may have caused the Black Plague, the *Variola* virus, and the Malaria protozoa) have been responsible for massive numbers of casualties and have had numerous effects on afflicted groups. Of particular note in modern times is HIV, which is known to have infected several million humans globally, along with the Influenza virus. Today, while many medical advances have been made to safeguard against infection by pathogens, through the use of vaccination, antibiotics, and fungicide, pathogens continue to threaten human life. Social advances such as food safety, hygiene, and water treatment have reduced the threat from some pathogens. Not all pathogens are negative. In entomology, pathogens are one of the "Three P's" (predators, pathogens, and parasitoids) that serve as natural or introduced biological controls to suppress arthropod pest populations.

Types of Pathogen

Viral: Pathogenic viruses are mainly those of the families of: Adenoviridae, Picornaviridae, Herpesviridae, Hepadnaviridae, Flaviviridae, Retroviridae, Orthomyxoviridae, Paramyxoviridae, Papovaviridae, Polyomavirus, Rhabdoviridae, Togaviridae. Some notable pathogenic viruses cause: smallpox, influenza, mumps, measles, chickenpox, ebola, and rubella. Viruses typically range between 20-300 nanometers in length.

Bacterial: Although the vast majority of bacteria are harmless or beneficial, a few pathogenic bacteria can cause infectious diseases. The most common bacterial disease is tuberculosis, caused by the bacterium *Mycobacterium tuberculosis*, which affects about 2 million people mostly in sub-Saharan Africa. Pathogenic bacteria contribute to other globally important diseases, such as pneumonia, which can be caused by bacteria such as *Streptococcus* and *Pseudomonas*, and foodborne illnesses, which can be caused by bacteria such as *Shigella*, *Campylobacter* and *Salmonella*. Pathogenic bacteria also cause infections such as tetanus, typhoid fever, diphtheria, syphilis and Hansen's disease. Bacteria can often be killed by antibiotics. They typically range between 1-5 micrometers in length.

Fungal: Fungi comprise a eukaryotic kingdom of microbes that are usually saprophytes but can cause diseases in humans, animals and plants. Fungi are the most common cause of diseases in crops and other plants.

Life threatening fungal infections in humans most often occur in immunocompromised patients or vulnerable people with a weakened immune system, although fungi are common problems in the immunocompetent population as the causative agents of skin, nail or yeast infections. Most antibiotics that function on bacterial pathogens cannot be used to treat fungal infections due to the fact that fungi and their hosts both have eukaryotic cells. Most clinical fungicides belong to the azole group. The typical fungal spore size is 1-40 micrometer in length.

Other Parasites

Some eukaryotic organisms, such as protists and helminths, cause disease. One of the best known diseases caused by protists in the genus *Plasmodium* is malaria. These can range from 3-200 micrometers in length.

Prionic: Prions are infectious pathogens that do not contain nucleic acids. Prions are abnormal proteins whose presence causes some diseases such as scrapie, bovine spongiform encephalopathy (mad cow disease) and Creutzfeldt–Jakob disease.. The discovery of prion as a new class of pathogen has lead Stanley B. Prusiner to receive Nobel Prize in Physiology or Medicine in 1997.

Potency: One hypothesis regarding pathogens states that the longer a pathogen can survive outside of the body, the more dangerous it can be to a potential host. For example, the smallpox virus (*variola virus*) can survive outside the human body for approximately 885 days. It is also one of the most deadly pathogenic viruses, as it kills between 20-50% of the people it infects. The tuberculosis bacterium kills 1 in 5 of the people it infects, but only survives 244 days outside of its host. However, research into the basis of the ability of pathogens to cause disease provides evidence from multiple and diverse species of the existence of pathogenicity or virulence factors, encoded within the pathogens' genetic material, that facilitate microbes to cause disease.

In countries that have higher sanitation standards, pathogens cannot survive for as long outside of the human. This is seen as encouragement to mutations to the pathogen which would make it less deadly, as such mutations would allow the pathogen to survive in the host for longer periods of time.

Transmission: One of the primary pathways by which food or water become contaminated is from the release of untreated sewage into a drinking water supply or onto cropland, with the result that people who eat or drink contaminated sources become infected. In developing countries most sewage is discharged into the environment or on cropland; even in developed countries there are periodic system failures resulting in a sanitary sewer overflow.

Antimicrobial

An anti-microbial is a substance that kills or inhibits the growth of microorganisms such as bacteria, fungi, or protozoans. Antimicrobial drugs either kill microbes (microbiocidal) or prevent the growth of microbes (microbiostatic). Disinfectants are antimicrobial substances used on non-living objects or outside the body. The history of antimicrobials begins with the observations of Pasteur and Joubert, who discovered that one type of bacteria could prevent the growth of another. They did not know at that time that the reason one bacterium failed to grow was that the other bacterium was producing an antibiotic. Technically, antibiotics are only those substances that are produced by one microorganism that kill, or prevent the growth, of another microorganism. Of course, in today's common usage, the term antibiotic is used to refer to almost any drug that attempts to rid your body of a bacterial infection. Antimicrobials include not just antibiotics, but synthetically formed compounds as well.

The discovery of antimicrobials like penicillin and tetracycline paved the way for better health for millions around the world. Before penicillin became a viable medical treatment in the early 1940s, no true cure for gonorrhea, strep throat, or pneumonia existed. Patients with infected wounds often had to have a wounded limb removed, or face death from infection. Now, most of these infections can be cured easily with a short course of antimicrobials.

However, with the development of antimicrobials, microorganisms have adapted and become resistant to previous antimicrobial agents. The old antimicrobial technology was based either on poisons or heavy metals, which may not have killed the microbe completely, allowing the microbe survive, change, and become resistant to the poisons and/or heavy metals. Antimicrobial nanotechnology is a recent addition to the fight against disease causing organisms, replacing heavy metals and toxins and may some day be a viable alternative. Infections that are acquired during a hospital visit are called "hospital acquired infections" or nosocomial infections. Similarly, when the infectious disease is picked up in the non-hospital setting it is considered "community acquired".

Main Classes

Antibiotics: Antibiotics are generally used to treat bacterial infections. The toxicity to humans and other animals from antibiotics is generally considered to be low. However, prolonged use of certain antibiotics can decrease the number of gut flora, which can have a negative impact on health. Some recommend that, during or after prolonged antibiotic use, one should consume probiotics and eat reasonably to replace destroyed gut flora.

The term antibiotic originally described only those formulations derived from living organisms, but is now applied also to synthetic antimicrobials, such as the sulfonamides.

The discovery, development, and clinical use of antibiotics during the 20th century has decreased substantially the mortality from bacterial infections. The antibiotic era began with the pneumatic application of nitroglycerine drugs, followed by a "golden" period of discovery from about 1945 to 1970, when a number of structurally diverse, highly effective agents were discovered and developed. However, since 1980 the introduction of new antimicrobial agents for clinical use has declined, in part because of the enormous expense of developing and testing new drugs. Paralleled to this there has been an alarming increase in bacterial resistance to existing agents.

Antibiotics are among the most commonly used drugs. For example, 30% or more hospitalized patients are treated with one or more courses of antibiotic therapy. However, antibiotics are also among the drugs commonly misused by physicians, e.g. usage of antibiotic agents in viral respiratory tract infections. The inevitable consequence of widespread and injudicious use of antibiotics has been the emergence of antibiotic-resistant pathogens, resulting in a serious threat to global public health. The resistance problem demands that a renewed effort be made to seek antibacterial agents effective against pathogenic bacteria resistant to current antibiotics. One of the possible strategies towards this objective is the rational localization of bioactive phytochemicals.

Antivirals: Antiviral drugs are a class of medication used specifically for treating viral infections. Like antibiotics for bacteria, specific antivirals are used for specific viruses. Unlike most antibiotics, antiviral drugs do not destroy their target pathogen; instead they inhibit their development. Antiviral drugs are one class of antimicrobials, a larger group which also includes antibiotic, antifungal and antiparasitic drugs. They are relatively harmless to the host, and therefore can be used to treat infections. They should be distinguished from viricides, which are not medication but destroy virus particles.

Most of the antivirals now available are designed to help deal with HIV, herpes viruses (best known for causing cold sores and genital herpes, but actually causing a wide range of diseases), the hepatitis B and C viruses, which can cause liver cancer, and influenza A and B viruses. Researchers are working to extend the range of antivirals to other families of pathogens.

Designing safe and effective antiviral drugs is difficult, because viruses use the host's cells to replicate. This makes it difficult to find targets for the drug that would interfere with the virus without also harming the host organism's cells.

The emergence of antivirals is the product of a greatly expanded knowledge of the genetic and molecular function of organisms, allowing biomedical researchers to understand the structure and function of viruses, major advances in the techniques for finding new drugs, and the intense pressure placed on the medical profession to deal with the human immunodeficiency virus (HIV), the cause of the deadly acquired immunodeficiency syndrome (AIDS) pandemic.

Almost all anti-microbials, including anti-virals, are subject to drug resistance as the pathogens mutate over time, becoming less susceptible to the treatment. For instance, a recent study published in Nature Biotechnology emphasized the urgent need for augmentation of oseltamivir (Tamiflu) stockpiles with additional antiviral drugs including zanamivir (Relenza) based on an evaluation of the performance of these drugs in the scenario that the 2009 H1N1 'Swine Flu' neuraminidase (NA) were to acquire the tamiflu-resistance (His274Tyr) mutation which is currently widespread in seasonal H1N1 strains.

History: Through the mid- to late-20th century, medical science and practice included an array of effective tools, ranging from antiseptics to vaccines and antibiotics, but no drugs to treat viral infections. While vaccines were effective in preventing many viral diseases, they could not help once a viral infection set in. Prior to the development of antivirals, when someone contracted a virus, there was little that could be done other than treating the symptoms and waiting for the disease to run its course.

The first experimental antivirals were developed in the 1960s, mostly to deal with herpes viruses, and were found using traditional trial-and-error drug discovery methods. Researchers grew cultures of cells and infected them with the target virus. They then introduced chemicals into the cultures they thought were likely to inhibit viral activity, and observed whether the level of virus in the cultures rose or fell.

Chemicals that seemed to have an effect were selected for closer study. This was a very time-consuming, hit-or-miss procedure, and in the absence of a good knowledge of how the target virus worked, it was not efficient in discovering antivirals that were effective and had few side effects. It was not until the 1980s, when the full genetic sequences of viruses began to be unraveled, that researchers began to learn how viruses worked in detail, and exactly what chemicals were needed to thwart their reproductive cycle. Dozens of antiviral treatments are now available, and medical research is rapidly exploiting new knowledge and technology to develop more.

Virus Life Cycle: Viruses consist of a genome and sometimes a few enzymes stored in a capsule made of protein (called a capsid), and sometimes covered with a lipid layer (sometimes called an 'envelope'). Viruses cannot reproduce on their own, and instead propagate by subjugating a host cell to produce copies of themselves, thus producing the next generation.

Researchers working on such "rational drug design" strategies for developing antivirals have tried to attack viruses at every stage of their life cycles. Some species of mushrooms have been found to contain multiple antiviral chemicals with similar synergistic effects. Viral life cycles vary in their precise details depending on the species of virus, but they all share a general pattern:

- Attachment to a host cell.
- Release of viral genes and possibly enzymes into the host cell.
- Replication of viral components using host-cell machinery.
- Assembly of viral components into complete viral particles.
- Release of viral particles to infect new host cells.

Limitations of Vaccines: Vaccines bolster the body's immune system to better attack viruses in the "complete particle" stage, outside of the organism's cells. They traditionally consist of an attenuated (weakened or killed) version of the virus. These vaccines can, in rare cases, harm the host by inadvertently infecting the host with a full-blown viral occupancy. Recently "subunit" vaccines have been devised that consist strictly of protein targets from the pathogen. They stimulate the immune system without doing serious harm to the host. In either case, when the real pathogen attacks the subject, the immune system responds to it quickly and blocks it. Vaccines are very effective on stable viruses, but are of limited use in treating a patient who has already been infected. They are also difficult to successfully deploy against rapidly mutating viruses, such as influenza (the vaccine for which is updated every year) and HIV. Antiviral drugs are particularly useful in these cases.

Anti-viral Targeting

The general idea behind modern antiviral drug design is to identify viral proteins, or parts of proteins, that can be disabled. These "targets" should generally be as unlike any proteins or parts of proteins in humans as possible, to reduce the likelihood of side effects. The targets should also be common across many strains of a virus, or even among different species of virus in the same family, so a single drug will have broad effectiveness. For example, a researcher might target a critical enzyme synthesized by the virus, but not the patient, that is common across strains, and see what can be done to interfere with its operation. Once targets are identified, candidate drugs can be selected, either from drugs already known to have appropriate effects, or by actually designing the candidate at the molecular level with a computer-aided design program. The target proteins can be manufactured in the lab for testing with candidate treatments by inserting the gene that synthesizes the target protein into bacteria or other kinds of cells. The cells are then cultured for mass production of the protein, which can then be exposed to various treatment candidates and evaluated with "rapid screening" technologies.

Approaches by Life Cycle Stage

Before Cell Entry: One anti-viral strategy is to interfere with the ability of a virus to infiltrate a target cell. The virus must go through a sequence of steps to do this, beginning with binding to a specific "receptor" molecule on the surface of the host cell and ending with the virus "uncoating" inside the cell and releasing its contents. Viruses that have a lipid envelope must also fuse their envelope with the target cell, or with a vesicle that transports them into the cell, before they can uncoat. This stage of viral replication can be inhibited in two ways:

- Using agents which mimic the virus-associated protein (VAP) and bind to the cellular receptors. This may include VAP anti-idiotypic antibodies, natural ligands of the receptor and anti-receptor antibodies.

- Using agents which mimic the cellular receptor and bind to the VAP. This includes anti-VAP antibodies, receptor anti-idiotypic antibodies, extraneous receptor and synthetic receptor mimics.

This strategy of designing drugs can be very expensive, and since the process of generating anti-idiotypic antibodies is partly trial and error, it can be a relatively slow process until an adequate molecule is produced.

Entry Inhibitor: A very early stage of viral infection is viral entry, when the virus attaches to and enters the host cell. A number of "entry-inhibiting" or "entry-blocking" drugs are being developed to fight HIV. HIV most heavily targets the immune system's white blood cells known as "helper T cells", and identifies these target cells through T-cell surface receptors designated "CD4" and "CCR5". Attempts to interfere with the binding of HIV with the CD4 receptor have failed to stop HIV from infecting helper T cells, but research continues on trying to interfere with the binding of HIV to the CCR5 receptor in hopes that it will be more effective.

Uncoating Inhibitor: Inhibitors of uncoating have also been investigated.

Amantadine and rimantadine, have been introduced to combat influenza. These agents act on penetration/uncoating. Pleconaril works against rhinoviruses, which cause the common cold, by blocking a pocket on the surface of the virus that controls the uncoating process. This pocket is similar in most strains of rhinoviruses and enteroviruses, which can cause diarrhea, meningitis, conjunctivitis, and encephalitis.

During Viral Synthesis

A second approach is to target the processes that synthesize virus components after a virus invades a cell.

Reverse Transcription

One way of doing this is to develop nucleotide or nucleoside analogues that look like the building blocks of RNA or DNA, but deactivate the enzymes that synthesize the RNA or DNA once the analogue is incorporated. This approach is more commonly associated with the inhibition of reverse transcriptase (RNA to DNA) than with "normal" transcriptase (DNA to RNA).

The first successful antiviral, acyclovir, is a nucleoside analogue, and is effective against herpesvirus infections. The first antiviral drug to be approved for treating HIV, zidovudine (AZT), is also a nucleoside analogue.

An improved knowledge of the action of reverse transcriptase has led to better nucleoside analogues to treat HIV infections. One of these drugs, lamivudine, has been approved to treat hepatitis B, which uses reverse transcriptase as part of its replication process. Researchers have gone further and developed inhibitors that do not look like nucleosides, but can still block reverse transcriptase.

Another target being considered for HIV antivirals include RNase H- which is a component of reverse transcriptase that splits the synthesized DNA from the original viral RNA.

Integrase

Another target is integrase, which splices the synthesized DNA into the host cell genome.

Transcription

Once a virus genome becomes operational in a host cell, it then generates messenger RNA (mRNA) molecules that direct the synthesis of viral proteins. Production of mRNA is initiated by proteins known as transcription factors. Several antivirals are now being designed to block attachment of transcription factors to viral DNA.

Translation/Antisense

Genomics has not only helped find targets for many antivirals, it has provided the basis for an entirely new type of drug, based on "antisense" molecules. These are segments of DNA or RNA that are designed as complementary molecule to critical sections of viral genomes, and the binding of these antisense segments to these target sections blocks the operation of those genomes. A phosphorothioate antisense drug named fomivirsen has been introduced, used to treat opportunistic eye infections in AIDS patients caused by cytomegalovirus, and other antisense antivirals are in development. An antisense structural type that has proven especially valuable in research is morpholino antisense.

Morpholino oligos have been used to experimentally suppress many viral types:

- caliciviruses
- flaviviruses (including WNV)
- dengue

- HCV
- coronaviruses.

Translation/Ribozymes

Yet another antiviral technique inspired by genomics is a set of drugs based on ribozymes, which are enzymes that will cut apart viral RNA or DNA at selected sites. In their natural course, ribozymes are used as part of the viral manufacturing sequence, but these synthetic ribozymes are designed to cut RNA and DNA at sites that will disable them. A ribozyme antiviral to deal with hepatitis C has been suggested, and ribozyme antivirals are being developed to deal with HIV. An interesting variation of this idea is the use of genetically modified cells that can produce custom-tailored ribozymes. This is part of a broader effort to create genetically modified cells that can be injected into a host to attack pathogens by generating specialized proteins that block viral replication at various phases of the viral life cycle.

Protease Inhibitors

Some viruses include an enzyme known as a protease that cuts viral protein chains apart so they can be assembled into their final configuration. HIV includes a protease, and so considerable research has been performed to find "protease inhibitors" to attack HIV at that phase of its life cycle. Protease inhibitors became available in the 1980s and have proven effective, though they can have unusual side effects, for example causing fat to build up in unusual places. Improved protease inhibitors are now in development. Protease inhibitors have also been seen in nature. A protease inhibitor was isolated from the Shiitake mushroom (*Lentinus edodes*). The presence of this may explain the Shiitake mushrooms noted antiviral activity *in vitro*.

Assembly

Rifampicin acts at the assembly phase.

Release Phase

The final stage in the life cycle of a virus is the release of completed viruses from the host cell, and this step has also been targeted by antiviral drug developers. Two drugs named zanamivir (Relenza) and oseltamivir (Tamiflu) that have been recently introduced to treat influenza prevent the release of viral particles by blocking a molecule named neuraminidase that is found on the surface of flu viruses, and also seems to be constant across a wide range of flu strains.

Immune System Stimulation

A second category of tactics for fighting viruses involves encouraging the body's immune system to attack them, rather than attacking them directly. Some antivirals of this sort do not focus on a specific pathogen, instead stimulating the immune system to attack a range of pathogens.

One of the best-known of this class of drugs are interferons, which inhibit viral synthesis in infected cells. One form of human interferon named "interferon alpha" is well-established as part of the standard treatment for hepatitis B and C, and other interferons are also being investigated as treatments for various diseases.

A more specific approach is to synthesize antibodies, protein molecules that can bind to a pathogen and mark it for attack by other elements of the immune system. Once researchers identify a particular target on the pathogen, they can synthesize quantities of identical "monoclonal" antibodies to link up that target. A monoclonal drug is now being sold to help fight respiratory syncytial virus in babies, and antibodies purified from infected individuals are also used as a treatment for hepatitis B.

Antifungals

An antifungal drug is medication used to treat fungal infections such as athlete's foot, ringworm, candidiasis (thrush), serious systemic infections such as cryptococcal meningitis, and others.

Antifungals work by exploiting differences between mammalian and fungal cells to kill off the fungal organism without dangerous effects on the host. Unlike bacteria, both fungi and humans are eukaryotes. Thus, fungal and human cells are similar at the molecular level, making it more difficult to find a target for an antifungal drug to attack that does not also exist in the infected organism. Consequently, there are often side effects to some of these drugs. Some of these side effects can be life-threatening if the drug is not used properly.

Antimicrobials and Home Mold remediation- Anti-fungal treatments are frequently sought-after to treat mold growth in damp or wetted home materials that exhibit mold growth. Note that most home mold problems are moisture/water-caused and the solution for conquering the mold growth is most dependent upon the water/moisture control and removal/discarding of the mold-damaged materials. Cleaning mold-damaged materials may result in a visually acceptable appearance but most cleaning methods kill mold or prevent its return.

For this reason, moisture management is the primary focus for mold prevention. Generally, Relative Humidity levels in the home above 54% will support mold groth on most cellulose containing materials (fabrics, carpeting and carpet backing, wood, paper, boxes, dust and lint). Mold also readily grows on most latex paints and leather. Antimicrobials used in home remediation follow a variety of chemistry and functions.

One common method of mold remediation utilizes Sodium Bicarbonate (Baking soda) as a blasting medium much in the way that sand is used to blast (clean) surfaces under the propulsion of compressed air. This 'Soda Blasting' makes a large cloud of dust that is pH Alkalai and its residue that permeates the wood and painted surfaces is also naturally antimicrobial as a result of the high pH and the presence of Sodium Bicarbonate. If used alone, repeated wetting can wash away the Sodium Bicarbonate residue and mold can return to the materials if the water source is not managed. Dry ice (frozen Carbon Dioxide (CO2)) is also used as a blasting agent where clean-up is more restrictive (i.e. attics) and while the dry ice blasting leaves no antimicrobial residue, it does prep the blasted surface to receive one as a secondary step.

One popular, professional anti-microbial (Serum) is often applied after or without blasting by soda or dry ice and in one of its variants, is a mix of Hydrogen Peroxide and thin surface coating that neutralizes the mold (making it non-viable) and encapsulating the surface to prevent spore release. Other anti-microbial surface treatments typically contain variants of metals known to supress mold grwoth; i.e. pigments or solutions involving Copper, Silver, Zinc or other metals (some of which can be toxic to humans if improperly applied). Most antimicrobial solutions are professionally applied and are not sold to the public.

Many people use either white vinegar or laundry bleach as an inexpensive anti-microbial solution. These liquids are best used in combination and they can be safely combined. When combined in equal amounts (i.e. 2 cups bleach + 2 cups vinegar in 2 gallons of warm water + 2 drops of dish soap), these make a solution known as "Acidified Bleach" and it is considerably more effective as an antimicroboial and as a disinfectant.

On porous foundation surfaces, a secondary step of scrubbing with Tri-Sodium Phosphate (TSP) or Spic-N-Span is capable of leaving behind a phosphate or carbonate reside that will be antimicrobial. The key to successful foundation cleaning with longer-lasting results hinges on leaving the cleaner residue on the wall and force-drying the area with a fan to drive off the water. Long-term success requires that the water source be corrected and that the area's relative humiidity be kept as far below 54% as possible. Antimicrobials and paints- Kitchen and Bath paint formulations are often manufactured with the understanding that these areas are often cleaned and may experience elevated humidity levels from bathing/cooking.

As a result, leading manufacturers often design Kitchen and Bath formulations to be less porous, more scrubable, and often, the paint formulation is adjusted to be more antimicrobial than other interior paints.

During colour mixing, some stores also offer the option of buying and adding an antimicrobial packet to the paint as a booster. It is ill-advised to use a normal latex paint on a foundation since this naturally moist area will readily cause mold to grow on latex. Foundation painting should be done with products designed for that purpose and when applied over virgin masonry, these products (i.e. DryLok by United Gilsonite Labs) perform very well.

Antiparasitics

Antiparasitics are a class of medications which are indicated for the treatment of infection by parasites, such as nematodes, cestodes, trematodes, infectious protozoa, and amoebae. Like antifungals, they must kill the infecting pest without serious damage to the host.

Non-pharmaceutical Antimicrobials

A wide range of chemical and natural compounds are used as antimicrobials. Organic acids are used widely as antimicrobials in food products, e.g. lactic acid, citric acid, acetic acid, and their salts, either as ingredients, or as disinfectants. For example, beef carcasses often are sprayed with acids, and then rinsed or steamed, to reduce the prevalence of E. coli O157:H7.

Traditional healers long have used plants to prevent or cure infectious disease. Many of these plants have been investigated scientifically for antimicrobial activity, and a large number of plant products have been shown to inhibit the growth of pathogenic microorganisms. A number of these agents appear to have structures and modes of action that are distinct from those of the antibiotics in current use, suggesting that cross-resistance with agents already in use may be minimal. So, it is worthwhile to study plants and plant products for activity against resistant bacteria.

Essential Oils

The antimicrobial properties of 21 plant essential oils and two essences were investigated against five food-borne pathogens, *Campylobacter jejuni, Salmonella enteriditis, Escherichia coli, Staphylococus aureus and Listeria monocytogenes*. The oils of bay, cinnamon, clove and thyme were the most inhibitory, each having a bacteriostatic concentration of 0.075% or less against all five pathogens. (A. Smith-Palmer, J. Stewart and L. Fyfe. Antimicrobial properties of plant essential oils and essences against five important food-borne pathogens. Letters in Applied Microbiology 1998. 26. 118-122)

Many essential oils are included in pharmacopoeias as having antimicrobial activity, including:

- Sideritis or Greek Mountain Tea
- Oregano oil
- Tea tree oil- in cosmetics, medicine
- Mint oil- in medicine, cosmetics (tooth paste etc.)
- Sandalwood oil- in cosmetics
- Clove oil- stomatology etc.
- Nigella sativa (Black cumin) oil
- Onion oil (*Allium cepe*)- phytoncides, in phytotherapy
- Leleshwa oil
- Lavender oil
- Lemon oil
- Lemon myrtle oil
- Neem oil
- Garlic
- Eucalyptus oil
- Peppermint oil
- Cinnamon oil
- Thyme oil.

Cations and Elements

Many heavy metal cations such as Hg^{2+}, Cu^{2+}, and Pb^{2+} have antimicrobial activities, but are also very toxic to other living organisms, thus making them unsuitable for treating infectious diseases. Colloidal silver is commonly used as an antimicrobial in alternative medicine without clear scientific proof of effectiveness.

Important Antibiotics and their Applications

Antibiotics are substances that inhibit the growth of microorganisms (anti- metabolites) or their replication (a bacteriostatic effect). They were traditionally obtained by extracting them from cultures of microbes. However, most drugs on the market today are semisynthetic derivatives of natural products. Sulfa drugs, discovered in the 1980s, were the first antimicrobial agents put into clinical use. Unfortunately, many bacteria are not susceptible to sulfonamides, and with the outbreak of World War II came the need for other more potent antibacterial agents. The serendipitous discovery of penicillin is, without a doubt, the most celebrated breakthrough in the history of antibiotics. In the late 1920s, while working in a London hospital, Alexander Fleming observed a mold overtaking a culture of staphylococcus bacteria he was growing in his laboratory. He extracted juices from the mold and, in 1929, reported that the extract, which he called penicillin, had antiseptic (anti-infectious) activity. The fungus was subsequently identified as *Penicillium notatum* (now called *Penicillium chrysogenum)*. It was not until the 1940s that penicillin was put into clinical use. Howard W. Florey, professor of pathology at Oxford's Sir William Dunn School of Pathology, and Ernst B. Chain are credited with culturing the fungus and producing the first significant quantities of penicillin for treating bacterial infections. In 1945 Fleming, Florey, and Chain received the Nobel Prize in physiology or medicine "for the discovery of penicillin and its curative effect in various infectious diseases."

Extracts from microorganisms are still an important source of antibiotics today. Clinically, antibiotics are described as possessing either broad- or narrow-spectrum activity. Bacteria are classified based on a staining technique developed by Danish microbiologist Hans Christian Gram. The bacterial cell walls of gram-positive bacteria stain blue when treated with either crystal violet or methylene blue, while gram-negative bacteria do not retain the stain and appear red. Broad-spectrum antibiotics are capable of inhibiting both gram-positive and gram-negative bacterial cultures. Grampositive bacteria have simpler cell walls than gram-negative strains and are susceptible to less toxic, narrow-spectrum antibiotics.

β-*Lactam Antibiotics*

A variety of penicillins have been produced by the fermentation of *Penicillium chrysogenum* in the presence of different nutrients. Penicillin G predominates when the culture medium is rich in phenylacetic acid, whereas the incorporation of phenoxyacetic acid favours penicillin V (phenoxymethylpenicillin). Semisynthetic penicillins, such as ampicillin and amoxicillin, are prepared by replacing the aromatic side chain of biosynthetically derived penicillins with other chemical groups. All penicillins are β-lactam antibiotics and have the same mechanism of action: They inhibit bacterial cell wall biosynthesis.

Bacterial cell walls differ from mammalian cell walls and are therefore attractive targets for antibiotics. Bacterial cell walls contain β-lactam receptors, known as penicillin-binding proteins (PBPs). β-Lactam antibiotics bind to the PBPs of bacterial cell walls and prevent their growth and repair. Widespread use of penicillin, however, has led to drug resistance. Because microorganisms multiply rapidly, strains of bacteria with enzymes capable of hydrolyzing β-lactam rings (β-lactamases) have evolved. β-lactamases are capable of inactivating β-lactam antibiotics before they bind to receptors on cell walls. As a result, physicians sometimes prescribe β-lactamase inhibitors to patients on penicillin therapy to circumvent drug inactivation by bacterial enzymes.

The cephalosporins comprise another important class of broad-spectrum β-lactam antibiotics. Cephalosporins were originally isolated from cultures of *Cephalosporium acremonium*. Cephalexin (Keflex) is a semisynthetic cephalosporin frequently prescribed to treat ear and skin infections caused by staphylococci or streptococci.

Antibiotics that Inhibit Protein Synthesis

There are also a large number of antibiotics structurally unrelated to penicillins and cephalosporins. These compounds exert their antimicrobial activity by inhibiting protein biosynthesis. In 1947 chloramphenicol was isolated from cultures of *Streptomyces venezuelae*. It is a broad-spectrum bacteriostatic agent that interferes with protein synthesis by binding to bacterial ribosomes. The use of chloramphenicol in humans is limited because of the drug's toxicity. It inhibits liver enzymes and suppresses red blood cell formation.

Aminoglycosides are amino sugars with broad-spectrum antibiotic activity. Streptomycin, isolated from *Streptomyces griseus,* was the first aminoglycoside antibiotic discovered. Although streptomycin initially proved to be a potent agent against gram-negative bacteria, rapid microbial resistance to the drug has limited its use and today streptomycin is generally administered in combination with other antibiotics. Neomycin is a broad-spectrum aminoglycoside antibiotic isolated from *Streptomyces fradiae.* However, because of the adverse effects of neomycin on the kidneys and ear, its use in humans is restricted to topical applications, often in combination with other antibiotics or corticosteroids. Concerns over the potential risks associated with aminoglycoside therapy, chiefly nephrotoxicity (kidney disease) and ototoxicity (damage to the ear canal), have diminished their use.

In 1952 the broad-spectrum antibiotic erythromycin was isolated from cultures of *Streptomyces erythreus* (later renamed *Saccharopolyspora erythraea).* The erythromycins are macrolide antibiotics that typically have a 12-, 14-, or 16-membered cyclic backbone which is a lactone.

Erythromycin A, the major fermentation component of *S. erythraea,* is a 14-membered ring macrolide that is used by medicinal chemists as the foundation for building semisynthetic derivatives of erythromycin antibiotics. (Macrolides inhibit bacteria by interfering with microbial protein biosynthesis.) Semisynthetic macrolides are popular with clinicians because they can be administered orally and have relatively low toxicity. They are often used to treat respiratory tract infections, and have been especially effective against conditions such as Legionnaires' disease and communityacquired pneumonia. Erythromycin therapy is often prescribed for individuals allergic to penicillin. One of the most widely used macrolide antibiotics derived from erythromycin A is azithromycin (Zithromax). Resistance to macrolide antibiotics generally involves mutations of bacterial ribosomal RNA that prevent macrolide binding.

In the late 1940s and early 1950s a series of tetracycline antibiotics was isolated from cultures of streptomyces. All tetracyclines consist of four fused 6-membered rings. Tetracyclines are broad-spectrum antibiotics that interfere with protein synthesis by binding to bacterial ribosomes. Unfortunately, the frequent use of tetracyclines to treat minor infections has led to resistance among previously susceptible strains of bacteria (pneumococci and staphylococci). Resistance to tetracyclines occurs when bacteria either develop proteins that prevent ribosomal binding by tetracyclines, or synthesize enzymes capable of inactivating tetracyclines.

Widespread use of antibiotics and rapid microbial evolution have led to highly resistant bacterial strains. Although most scientists no longer believe that a single drug will be developed to wipe out all infectious diseases, there is increasing demand for new antimicrobial agents. Currently, combined drug therapy appears to be the most effective means of circumventing microbial resistance to antibiotics.

P Enicillin

Penicillin was discovered accidentally in 1929 when Sir Alexander Fleming observed bacterial cultures contaminated with a mold that inhibited bacterial growth. The antibiotic penicillin was subsequently isolated from cultures of the *Penicillium* mold. In 1938 two other British scientists, Howard Florey and Ernst Chain, first used purified preparations of penicillin to treat bacterial infections. Penicillin may have been present in folk remedies used as early as 600 B.C.E., at around which time molded soybean curd was used by the Chinese to treat boils and carbuncles, and moldy cheese was used by Chinese and Ukrainian peasants to treat infected wounds.

Initially it was thought that penicillin was a pure substance, but further studies revealed that a number of closely related compounds were present in *Penicillium* cultures. Naturally occurring penicillins, such as penicillin G, are most effective against gram-positive bacteria, but much less effective against gram-negative bacteria. A further limitation to the use of Penicillin G is that it is not well absorbed when administered orally. Research programs to produce chemically modified penicillins with improved properties have resulted in a large number of clinically useful penicillin derivatives. Examples of such penicillin derivatives include ampicillin and amoxicillin, which have much greater efficacy against gram-negative bacteria than penicillin, retain good activity against gram-positive bacteria, and are well absorbed when administered orally. The principal adverse reaction associated with the penicillins is the occurrence of allergic response.

The molecular targets for the antibacterial activity of the penicillin and related β-lactam antibiotics such as the cephalosporins are a group of bacterial enzymes known as *penicillin-binding proteins* (PBPs). The PBPs are essential to the final stages of bacterial cell wall biosynthesis. Penicillin and other β-lactam antibiotics inhibit PBPs, thereby inhibiting bacterial cell wall biosynthesis, which eventually results in bacterial cell lysis. (Vancomycin and cycloserine are nonpenicillin antibiotics that also inhibit bacterial cell wall biosynthesis through other mechanisms.) The penicillins and related antibiotics have been among the most widely used therapeutic agents since their introduction into clinical practice in the 1940s. However, the widespread use of these antibiotics has resulted in the emergence and spread of bacteria that are resistant to these agents. A major mechanism of resistance to the penicillin and other β-lactam antibiotics is the bacterial production of β-lactamases, enzymes that cleave the β-lactam antibiotics and render them inactive before they can inhibit their PBP targets. Significant efforts have been made to develop β-lactam antibiotics resistant to the β-lactamases, and toward finding inhibitors of the β-lactamases to allow β-lactam antibiotics to be useful antibacterial agents against β-lactamase producing bacteria.

Gram-positive and Gram-negative Bacteria

Bacteria can be broadly classified into two groups; the gram-positive bacteria, which are stained purple after the gram staining procedure, and the gram-negative bacteria, which are stained red. The difference in staining reflects differences in the structure of the cell walls between gram-positive and gram-negative bacteria. Pathogenic gram-positive bacteria include Staphylococcus aureus and Bacillus anthracis, and pathogenic gram-negative bacteria include Escherichia coli and Neisseria gonorrhoeae.

S Ulfa D Rugs

Sulfa drugs were the first synthetic drugs with widespread antibiotic activity to be put into clinical use. In the 1930s German chemists observed that certain dyes used to stain bacteria stopped microbial growth. Gerhard Domagk, a pathologist at I. G. Farbenindustrie, performed a series of experiments on mice infected with streptococcus bacteria and observed that mice injected with an orange-red dye called Prontosil survived bacterial infection. Prontosil is an azo dye that had not shown antibacterial activity during earlier in vitro tests. However, in vivo, the dye is transformed into sulfanilamide, a compound with antimicrobial activity. Domagk had such faith in Prontosil's anti-infectious properties that he is reported to have injected the dye into his daughter when she had septicemia. In 1939 Domagk was awarded the Nobel Prize in physiology or medicine for his discovery.

Once sulfanilamide was recognized as an active antimicrobial agent, scientists synthesized thousands of sulfonamides to test for bactericidal activity. It was later realized that sulfonamides do not actually kill bacteria; they interfere with bacterial growth and replication. Sulfa drugs are bacteriostatic. They inhibit an enzyme necessary for the biosynthesis of folic acid in bacteria. Folic acid is necessary for the biosynthesis of thymine and the purine bases, the building blocks of DNA. Bacteria that are sensitive to sulfa drugs are unable to acquire folic acid from their environment and, in the presence of sulfonamides, are unable to synthesize the folic acid essential for cell growth and multiplication. Sulfonamides do not harm their human hosts, however, because, unlike susceptible bacteria, humans acquire folic acid from their diet and lack the enzyme necessary for synthesizing folic acid.

Production of Penicillin

Many fungal species grow on food products, often contributing to their spoilage, as in fruits, vegetables, and other fresh or prepared products. However, in many instances the presence of fungi on some products does not have a deleterious effect and may even contribute to the ripening and development of important organoleptic characteristics typical of a particular food (17, 19). This is the case of fungi belonging to the genus *Penicillium*, which grow on cured meat products and on many kinds of cheese. Some of these fungi whose presence is beneficial for the product are nowadays used as starters, as a means to colonize homogeneously the cheese or meat piece, thus preventing the eventual colonization by undesirable fungi and bacteria.

Some of the fungal species most widely used as starters are *Penicillium nalgiovense* and *Penicillium chrysogenum* for meat products, *Penicillium roqueforti* for Roquefort cheese, and *Penicillium camemberti* for Camembert cheese. Most fungi growing on food are producers of mycotoxins and antibiotics (28, 39, 46), and the presence of the compounds secreted by the fungus in the colonized food product has been reported on different occasions (9, 31). Laich et al. (25) showed that *P. nalgiovense* produces penicillin on the surface of a Spanish fermented sausage (fuet); the presence of the antibiotic can be detected in the outer layers of the sausages.

The presence of penicillin in food is not desirable, as it can produce allergic reactions (18, 20, 29) and might eventually lead to the development of resistance phenomena in human resident bacteria, which could then transfer that genetic information to pathogenic bacteria, as resistance gene transfer between bacteria in the human colon has been shown to be a common phenomenon (42). The development of resistance phenomena in bacteria as a consequence of the ingestion of subtherapeutic levels of antibiotics has been reported in several cases in farm animals (1, 34).

Therefore, it is important to know whether fungi associated with food production are potential penicillin producers or not. The objective of the present work was to analyse the possible production of penicillin and to study the presence of the penicillin biosynthetic genes in fungi of the genus *Penicillium* growing on food products or used as starters for those products.

Materials and Methods

Penicillium Strains

Some of the fungal species were chosen for the present study because they are commonly used as commercial starters (*P. nalgiovense*, *P. chrysogenum*, *P. camemberti*, and *P. roqueforti*); the rest of the species were chosen because of their frequent isolation from cured meat products like cecina (a salted and smoked-cured beef meat product from north Spain) as part of the natural mycobiota growing on this product (F. Laich, F. Fierro, and J. F. Martín, unpublished results).

P. chrysogenum NRRL 1951; *P. nalgiovense* NRRL 911; *Penicillium griseofulvum* NRRL 2300, NRRL 2152, NRRL 989, NRRL 994, NRRL 991, and NRRL 992; *P. roqueforti* NRRL 849; *P. camemberti* NRRL 874, NRRL 877, NRRL 876 (ex-type of *Penicillium candidum*), and CECT 2267; *Penicillium verrucosum* NRRL 5573 and NRRL 5574; *Penicillium brevicompactum* NRRL 862; *Penicillium commune* NRRL 845; *Penicillium solitum* NRRL 937; *Penicillium crustosum* NRRL 972; *Penicillium expansum* NRRL 976; *Penicillium implicatum* NRRL 2061; *Penicillium hirsutum* NRRL 2032; *Penicillium aurantiogriseum* NRRL 971; *Penicillium viridicatum* NRRL 963; *Penicillium echinulatum* NRRL 1151; *Penicillium purpurogenum* ATCC MYA-38; and *Paecilomyces variotii* NRRL 1775 were obtained either from the ARS Culture Collection (Peoria, Ill.), the American Type Culture Collection (ATCC) (Manassas, Va.), or the Spanish type culture collection (CECT) (Valencia, Spain).

Other strains were isolated from cheese (inner part) and cecina (surface) as indicated by Motilva Casado et al.. For colony isolation, samples were plated on malt extract agar (MEA) and incubated at 25°C for 7 days. The strains isolated were identified to species level according to the method of Pitt and Hocking and genetic analysis. Once the strains were identified they were named as follows: *P. nalgiovense* 16a, *P. commune* INBCC300, and *P. chrysogenum* AK (all isolated from cecina); and *P. roqueforti* CONT1 (isolated from blue cheese).

P. chrysogenum AS-P-78 was kindly donated by Antibióticos, S.A. (León, Spain). *P. nalgiovense* INBCC103 is a commercial starter culture.

Identification Procedures

All isolates were identified to the species level according to the method of Pitt and Hocking. To confirm this identification, the randomly amplified polymorphic DNA (RAPD) technique was used. Total DNA was obtained as described by Fierro et al. RAPD PCR amplification was carried out according to the protocol described by Williams et al. with modifications. PCRs were performed with a 25-µl volume containing the following: 16 mM $(NH_4)_2SO_4$; 67 mM Tris-HCl, pH 8.8; 0.01% Tween 20; 3.5 mM $MgCl_2$; a 200 µM concentration (each) of dATP, dCTP, dGTP, and dTTP (Fermentas); 0.32 µM primer; 0.5 U of *Taq* DNA polymerase (Bioline); and 10 to 20 ng of genomic DNA. The following oligonucleotides were used: 1, 5'-AGTCAGCCAC-3'; 2, 5'-AATCGGGCT-3'; CRL9, 5'-CAGCCGCCCC-3'; and CRL12, 5'-CCGCCGCCCG-3'. PCR was carried out with a Whatman Biometra T Gradient thermal cycler using an initial denaturation step of 94°C for 4 min; followed by 45 cycles of 40 s at 94°C, 1 min at 34°C, and 2 min at 72°C; and a final extension of 72°C for 10 min. Amplified fragments were separated on a 1.5% (wt/vol) agarose gel and visualized by ethidium bromide staining.

Bioassays for Penicillin Production

All the strains described above were tested for their ability to produce penicillin by bioassays in both solid and liquid medium with *Micrococcus luteus* ATCC 9341 as a test strain. ß-Lactamase from *Bacillus cereus* UL1 (300 µl from the supernatant of a *B. cereus* culture per 100 ml of tryptic soy agar [TSA] medium) was used to check if the antibacterial activity observed in the samples was due to the presence of penicillin or to some other antagonistic compound.

The bioassay on solid medium was performed by growing the fungus in petri dishes on MEA at 25°C for 7 to 10 days (when a high number of conidia was produced by the colony). Agar plugs (9-mm diameter) were taken out of the fungal colonies, placed on the surface of TSA medium (Difco) containing 1% agar, and incubated for 48 h at 25°C.

Then, an overlayer of 1% TSA with *M. luteus* was added onto the medium with the plugs, the antibiotic was allowed to diffuse in the plates in the cold (2 h at 5°C), and finally the cultures were incubated at 30°C for 24 h.

Studies of the production of penicillin on liquid cultures were carried out as described previously.

HPLC Analysis

P. griseofulvum NRRL 2300 was fermented on a liquid culture in CPM medium under the conditions described before. Samples from the supernatant were taken after 96 h of fermentation. Fifty microliters of both the unprocessed supernatant and an ethyl acetate-extracted fraction obtained as described previously by Laich et al. was analysed with a Waters high-performance liquid chromatograph (HPLC) with a μBondapak C_{18} column. Penicillin G at a concentration of 0.1 mg/ml was used as the control sample. Buffer A was 50 mM sodium acetate, pH 4.5, and buffer B was acetonitrile. The flow rate was 1.3 ml/min, and the running conditions were as follows: min 1 to 3, buffer A; min 3 to 15, gradient buffer B, 0 to 60%; min 15 to 18, gradient buffer B, 60 to 80%; min 18 to 20, buffer B, 80%; min 20 to 22, gradient buffer B, 80 to 0%; and min 22 to 25, buffer A.

Southern Blotting and Hybridization

Total DNA of the fungi was extracted as described before. Five micrograms of DNA of each strain was digested with the restriction endonuclease *Eco*RI. The DNA fragments were separated on a horizontal 0.6% agarose gel and transferred onto a Hybond-N membrane (Amersham Pharmacia Biotech) using a vacuum blotter (VacuGene XL; Pharmacia Biotech). The probes were labelled with the DIG DNA labeling mixture (Boehringer Mannheim) according to the manufacturer's protocol. Prehybridization and hybridization were done with 40% formamide standard buffer at 42°C.

After hybridization, the membrane was washed at room temperature for 15 min with 2x SSC (1x SSC is 0.15 M NaCl plus 0.015 M sodium citrate)-0.1% sodium dodecyl sulfate (SDS), 15 min at 42°C with 0.1x SSC-0.1% SDS, and 3 min at 65°C with 0.1x SSC-0.1% SDS. The signals were visualized with a chemiluminescent substrate for alkaline phosphatase (Roche) according to the manufacturer's protocol.

PCR Amplification and Sequencing

The letter code used for nucleotide designation is according to the Nomenclature Committee of the International Union of Biochemistry. PCR amplification was performed by standard procedures. In the case of primers PVCG and PVCB, an annealing temperature gradient between 46 and 69°C was used. DNA sequencing was performed with an ABI PRISM 310 Genetic Analyser (PE Applied Biosystems) using standard sequencing primers and the ABI PRISM sequencing kit, according to the manufacturer's instructions.

Results

Penicillin Production by Different Strains

All the strains were first screened to detect penicillin producers using a very sensitive bioassay in solid medium. No antibacterial activity was observed after five bioassays of strains belonging to the species *P. roqueforti*, *P. camemberti*, *P. brevicompactum*, *P. commune*, *P. solitum*, *P. expansum*, *P. implicatum*, *P. hirsutum*, *P. aurantiogriseum*, *P. viridicatum*, *P. echinulatum*, *P. purpurogenum*, and *Paecilomyces variotii*. However, strains belonging to *P. chrysogenum*, *P. nalgiovense*, *P. griseofulvum*, *P. crustosum*, and *P. verrucosum* consistently showed different levels of antibacterial activity. The highest antibacterial activity was found in *P. chrysogenum* AK, followed by *P. griseofulvum* NRRL 2300 and by *P. nalgiovense* 16a. ß-Lactamase from *B. cereus* UL1 was used as a means to discern between the antibacterial activity caused by penicillin and that exerted by other antagonistic substances that the fungus might produce. However, in three other strains of *P. griseofulvum* (NRRL 991, NRRL 992, and NRRL 989) only part of the antibacterial activity could be attributed to penicillin, as a smaller penicillinase-resistant inhibition halo was still formed in the presence of ß-lactamase.

In *P. verrucosum* and *P. crustosum*, no decrease of the inhibition halo was observed upon treatment with ß-lactamase, which indicates that the antibacterial activity observed in this case is not caused by penicillin but by some other compound(s).

Penicillin production by *P. griseofulvum* strains in solid medium was confirmed by fermentation in liquid submerged cultures. *P. griseofulvum* strain NRRL 2300 showed the highest production level, while the rest of the *P. griseofulvum* strains produced much smaller amounts (less than 10 μg/ml). In some of the strains, penicillin production was detected only after 80 h of fermentation.

An HPLC analysis of the supernatant of a *P. griseofulvum* NRRL 2300 liquid culture was performed to confirm that the antibiotic produced by this fungus was penicillin. It was, therefore, concluded that *P. griseofulvum* produces authentic penicillin G.

Analysis of the Presence of Penicillin Biosynthetic Genes in Different Strains

The results on production of penicillin observed in the previous experiments should correlate with the presence or absence of the penicillin biosynthetic genes *pcbAB*, *pcbC*, and *penDE* in the different strains. We performed a series of Southern blot analyses to detect the possible presence of the genes in all the strains used in this study. Probes C, D, and E correspond to the *pcbAB* gene, encoding L-- aminoadipyl-L-cysteinyl-D-valine (ACV) synthetase, the multidomain enzyme catalyzing the first step of the biosynthesis of penicillin. Probes A and B correspond to the *pcbC* and *penDE* genes, respectively, which encode the enzymes responsible for the second and third step of the biosynthesis. The results obtained with probes A and B indicate that both the *pcbC* and the *penDE* genes are present in all the strains of *P. chrysogenum*, *P. nalgiovense*, and *P. griseofulvum* and are absent in all the remaining strains belonging to other species. The presence of the penicillin gene cluster confirms that *P. griseofulvum* is a penicillin producer.

Similarly, the absence of the penicillin cluster in *P. verrucosum* and *P. crustosum* supports the conclusion that the antibacterial activity observed in these fungi is not due to penicillin. All the strains of *P. griseofulvum* contained the whole *pcbAB* gene, as revealed by the hybridization signals appearing with the three probes C, D, and E. The Southern blot analyses performed with these five probes, along with additional Southern blots with other probes from the cluster, allowed us to elaborate on an *Eco*RI restriction map of the new penicillin gene cluster in *P. griseofulvum* by comparison with the previously described maps of *P. chrysogenum* (6) and *P. nalgiovense* (25). There is an *Eco*RI site in the *penDE* gene of the *P. griseofulvum* NRRL 991 strain which is absent in the other strains of *P. griseofulvum*. In general most of the restriction sites are conserved between the three species, but it is striking that one of the *Eco*RI fragments inside *pcbAB* is about 160 bp larger in *P. griseofulvum* than in *P. chrysogenum*.

Chapter

7

Microbial Biodegradation

Bioremediation is the use of microorganismal metabolism to remove pollutants. Technologies can be generally classified as *in situ* or *ex situ*. *In situ* bioremediation involves treating the contaminated material at the site, while *ex situ* involves the removal of the contaminated material to be treated elsewhere. Some examples of bioremediation technologies are bioventing, landfarming, bioreactor, composting, bioaugmentation, rhizofiltration, and biostimulation.

Bioremediation can occur on its own (natural attenuation or intrinsic bioremediation) or can be spurred on via the addition of fertilizers to increase the bioavailability within the medium (biostimulation). Recent advancements have also proven successful via the addition of matched microbe strains to the medium to enhance the resident microbe population's ability to break down contaminants. Microorganisms used to perform the function of bioremediation are known as Bioremediators.(bioaugmentation).

Not all contaminants, however, are easily treated by bioremediation using microorganisms. For example, heavy metals such as cadmium and lead are not readily absorbed or captured by organisms. The assimilation of metals such as mercury into the food chain may worsen matters. Phytoremediation is useful in these circumstances because natural plants or transgenic plants are able to bioaccumulate these toxins in their above-ground parts, which are then harvested for removal. The heavy metals in the harvested biomass may be further concentrated by incineration or even recycled for industrial use. The elimination of a wide range of pollutants and wastes from the environment requires increasing our understanding of the relative importance of different pathways and regulatory networks to carbon flux in particular environments and for particular compounds, and they will certainly accelerate the development of bioremediation technologies and biotransformation processes.

Genetic Engineering Approaches

The use of genetic engineering to create organisms specifically designed for bioremediation has great potential. The bacterium *Deinococcus radiodurans* (the most radioresistant organism known) has been modified to consume and digest toluene and ionic mercury from highly radioactive nuclear waste.

Most commonly, the process is misunderstood. The microbes are ever-present in any given context and are generally referred to as "normal microbial flora". During bioremediation (biodegradation) processes, fertilizer/nutrient supplementation is introduced to the environments in efforts to maximize growth and production potential. Common misbelief is that microbes are transported and dispersed into an unadulterated environment.

Mycoremediation

Mycoremediation is a form of bioremediation in which fungi are used to decontaminate the area. The term *mycoremediation* refers specifically to the use of fungal mycelia in bioremediation. One of the primary roles of fungi in the ecosystem is decomposition, which is performed by the mycelium. The mycelium secretes extracellular enzymes and acids that break down lignin and cellulose, the two main building blocks of plant fibre. These are organic compounds composed of long chains of carbon and hydrogen, structurally similar to many organic pollutants. The key to mycoremediation is determining the right fungal species to target a specific pollutant. Certain strains have been reported to successfully degrade the nerve gases VX and sarin.

In one conducted experiment, a plot of soil contaminated with diesel oil was inoculated with mycelia of oyster mushrooms; traditional bioremediation techniques (bacteria) were used on control plots. After four weeks, more than 95% of many of the PAH (polycyclic aromatic hydrocarbons) had been reduced to non-toxic components in the mycelial-inoculated plots. It appears that the natural microbial community participates with the fungi to break down contaminants, eventually into carbon dioxide and water. Wood-degrading fungi are particularly effective in breaking down aromatic pollutants (toxic components of petroleum), as well as chlorinated compounds. Mycofiltration is a similar process, using fungal mycelia to filter toxic waste and microorganisms from water in soil.

Advantages

There are a number of cost/efficiency advantages to bioremediation, which can be employed in areas that are inaccessible without excavation. For example, hydrocarbon spills (specifically, petrol spills) or certain chlorinated solvents may contaminate groundwater, and introducing the appropriate electron acceptor or electron donor amendment, as appropriate, may significantly reduce contaminant concentrations after a long time allowing for acclimation. This is typically much less expensive than excavation followed by disposal elsewhere, incineration or other *ex situ* treatment strategies, and reduces or eliminates the need for "pump and treat", a practice common at sites where hydrocarbons have contaminated clean groundwater.

Monitoring Bioremediation

The process of bioremediation can be monitored indirectly by measuring the *Oxidation Reduction Potential* or redox in soil and groundwater, together with pH, temperature, oxygen content, electron acceptor/donor concentrations, and concentration of breakdown products (e.g. carbon dioxide). This table shows the (decreasing) biological breakdown rate as function of the redox potential.

Process	*Reaction*	*Redox potential (E_h in mV)*
aerobic:	$O_2 + 4e^- + 4H^+ \rightarrow 2H_2O$	600 ~ 400
anaerobic:		
denitrification	$2NO_3^- + 10e^- + 12H^+ \rightarrow N_2 + 6H_2O$	500 ~ 200
manganese IV reduction	$MnO_2 + 2e^- + 4H^+ \rightarrow Mn^{2+} + 2H_2O$	400 ~ 200
iron III reduction	$Fe(OH)_3 + e^- + 3H^+ \rightarrow Fe^{2+} + 3H_2O$	300 ~ 100
sulfate reduction	$SO_4^{2-} + 8e^- + 10H^+ \rightarrow H_2S + 4H_2O$	0 ~ –150
fermentation	$2CH_2O \rightarrow CO_2 + CH_4$	–150 ~ –220

This, by itself and at a single site, gives little information about the process of remediation.

1. It is necessary to sample enough points on and around the contaminated site to be able to determine contours of equal redox potential. Contouring is usually done using specialised software, e.g. using Kriging interpolation.

2. If all the measurements of redox potential show that electron acceptors have been used up, it is in effect an indicator for total microbial activity. Chemical analysis is also required to determine when the levels of contaminants and their breakdown products have been reduced to below regulatory limits.

Microbial Biodegradation

Interest in the microbial biodegradation of pollutants has intensified in recent years as humanity strives to find sustainable ways to cleanup contaminated environments. These bioremediation and biotransformation methods endeavour to harness the astonishing, naturally occurring, ability of microbial xenobiotic metabolism to degrade, transform or accumulate a huge range of compounds including hydrocarbons (e.g. oil), polychlorinated biphenyls (PCBs), polyaromatic hydrocarbons (PAHs), heterocyclic compounds (such as pyridine or quinoline), pharmaceutical substances, radionuclides and metals. Major methodological breakthroughs in recent years have enabled detailed genomic, metagenomic, proteomic, bioinformatic and other high-throughput analyses of environmentally relevant microorganisms providing unprecedented insights into key biodegradative pathways and the ability of organisms to adapt to changing environmental conditions.

The elimination of a wide range of pollutants and wastes from the environment is an absolute requirement to promote a sustainable development of our society with low environmental impact. Biological processes play a major role in the removal of contaminants and they take advantage of the astonishing catabolic versatility of microorganisms to degrade/convert such compounds. New methodological breakthroughs in sequencing, genomics, proteomics, bioinformatics and imaging are producing vast amounts of information. In the field of Environmental Microbiology, genome-based global studies open a new era providing unprecedented *in silico* views of metabolic and regulatory networks, as well as clues to the evolution of degradation pathways and to the molecular adaptation strategies to changing environmental conditions. Functional genomic and metagenomic approaches are increasing our understanding of the relative importance of different pathways and regulatory networks to carbon flux in particular environments and for particular compounds and they will certainly accelerate the development of bioremediation technologies and biotransformation processes.

Aerobic Biodegradation of Pollutants

The burgeoning amount of bacterial genomic data provides unparalleled opportunities for understanding the genetic and molecular bases of the degradation of organic pollutants. Aromatic compounds are among the most recalcitrant of these pollutants and lessons can be learned from the recent genomic studies of *Burkholderia xenovorans* LB400 and *Rhodococcus* sp. strain RHA1, two of the largest bacterial genomes completely sequenced to date. These studies have helped expand our understanding of bacterial catabolism, non-catabolic physiological adaptation to organic compounds, and the evolution of large bacterial genomes. First, the metabolic pathways from phylogenetically diverse isolates are very similar with respect to overall organization. Thus, as originally noted in pseudomonads, a large number of "peripheral aromatic" pathways funnel a range of natural and xenobiotic compounds into a restricted number of "central aromatic" pathways.

Nevertheless, these pathways are genetically organized in genus-specific fashions, as exemplified by the b-ketoadipate and Paa pathways. Comparative genomic studies further reveal that some pathways are more widespread than initially thought. Thus, the Box and Paa pathways illustrate the prevalence of non-oxygenolytic ring-cleavage strategies in aerobic aromatic degradation processes. Functional genomic studies have been useful in establishing that even organisms harboring high numbers of homologous enzymes seem to contain few examples of true redundancy. For example, the multiplicity of ring-cleaving dioxygenases in certain rhodococcal isolates may be attributed to the cryptic aromatic catabolism of different terpenoids and steroids. Finally, analyses have indicated that recent genetic flux appears to have played a more significant role in the evolution of some large genomes, such as LB400's, than others. However, the emerging trend is that the large gene repertoires of potent pollutant degraders such as LB400 and RHA1 have evolved principally through more ancient processes. That this is true in such phylogenetically diverse species is remarkable and further suggests the ancient origin of this catabolic capacity.

Anaerobic Biodegradation of Pollutants

Anaerobic microbial mineralization of recalcitrant organic pollutants is of great environmental significance and involves intriguing novel biochemical reactions. In particular, hydrocarbons and halogenated compounds have long been doubted to be degradable in the absence of oxygen, but the isolation of hitherto unknown anaerobic hydrocarbon-degrading and reductively dehalogenating bacteria during the last decades provided ultimate proof for these processes in nature. Many novel biochemical reactions were discovered enabling the respective metabolic pathways, but progress in the molecular understanding of these bacteria was rather slow, since genetic systems are not readily applicable for most of them. However, with the increasing application of genomics in the field of environmental microbiology, a new and promising perspective is now at hand to obtain molecular insights into these new metabolic properties. Several complete genome sequences were determined during the last few years from bacteria capable of anaerobic organic pollutant degradation. 4.7 Mb genome of the facultative denitrifying *Aromatoleum aromaticum* strain EbN1 was the first to be determined for an anaerobic hydrocarbon degrader (using toluene or ethylbenzene as substrates).

The genome sequence revealed about two dozen gene clusters (including several paralogs) coding for a complex catabolic network for anaerobic and aerobic degradation of aromatic compounds. The genome sequence forms the basis for current detailed studies on regulation of pathways and enzyme structures. Further genomes of anaerobic hydrocarbon degrading bacteria were recently completed for the iron-reducing species *Geobacter metallireducens* (accession nr. NC_007517) and the perchlorate-reducing *Dechloromonas aromatica* (accession nr. NC_007298), but these are not yet evaluated in formal publications.

Complete genomes were also determined for bacteria capable of anaerobic degradation of halogenated hydrocarbons by halorespiration: the ~1.4 Mb genomes of *Dehalococcoides ethenogenes* strain 195 and *Dehalococcoides* sp. strain CBDB1 and the ~5.7 Mb genome of *Desulfitobacterium hafniense* strain Y51. Characteristic for all these bacteria is the presence of multiple paralogous genes for reductive dehalogenases, implicating a wider dehalogenating spectrum of the organisms than previously known. Moreover, genome sequences provided unprecedented insights into the evolution of reductive dehalogenation and differing strategies for niche adaptation.

Recently, it has become apparent that some organisms, including *Desulfitobacterium chlororespirans*, originally evaluated for halorespiration on chlorophenols, can also use certain brominated compounds, such as the herbicide bromoxynil and its major metabolite as electron acceptors for growth. Iodinated compounds may be dehalogenated as well, though the process may not satisfy the need for an electron acceptor.

Bioavailability, Chemotaxis, and Transport of Pollutants

Bioavailability, or the amount of a substance that is physiochemically accessible to microorganisms is a key factor in the efficient biodegradation of pollutants. O'Loughlin et al (2000) showed that, with the exception of kaolinite clay, most soil clays and cation exchange resins attenuated biodegradation of 2-picoline by *Arthrobacter* sp. strain R1, as a result of adsorption of the substrate to the clays. Chemotaxis, or the directed movement of motile organisms towards or away from chemicals in the environment is an important physiological response that may contribute to effective catabolism of molecules in the environment. In addition, mechanisms for the intracellular accumulation of aromatic molecules via various transport mechanisms are also important.

Oil Biodegradation

Petroleum oil contains aromatic compounds that are toxic for most life forms. Episodic and chronic pollution of the environment by oil causes major ecological perturbations. Marine environments are especially vulnerable since oil spills of coastal regions and the open sea are poorly containable and mitigation is difficult. In addition to pollution through human activities, about 250 million litres of petroleum enter the marine environment every year from natural seepages. Despite its toxicity, a considerable fraction of petroleum oil entering marine systems is eliminated by the hydrocarbon-degrading activities of microbial communities, in particular by a remarkable recently discovered group of specialists, the so-called hydrocarbonoclastic bacteria (HCB). *Alcanivorax borkumensis* was the first HCB to have its genome sequenced. In addition to hydrocarbons, crude oil often contains various heterocyclic compounds, such as pyridine, which appear to be degraded by similar, though separate mechanisms than hydrocarbons.

Analysis of Waste Biotreatment

Sustainable development requires the promotion of environmental management and a constant search for new technologies to treat vast quantities of wastes generated by increasing anthropogenic activities. Biotreatment, the processing of wastes using living organisms, is an environmentally friendly, relatively simple and cost-effective alternative to physico-chemical clean-up options. Confined environments, such as bioreactors, have been engineered to overcome the physical, chemical and biological limiting factors of biotreatment processes in highly controlled systems. The great versatility in the design of confined environments allows the treatment of a wide range of wastes under optimized conditions. To perform a correct assessment, it is necessary to consider various microorganisms having a variety of genomes and expressed transcripts and proteins. A great number of analyses are often required. Using traditional genomic techniques, such assessments are limited and time-consuming. However, several high-throughput techniques originally developed for medical studies can be applied to assess biotreatment in confined environments.

Phyto-remediation

Phytoremediation, and Latin *remedium* (*restoring balance* or *remediation*) describes the treatment of environmental problems (bioremediation) through the use of plants that mitigate the environmental problem without the need to excavate the contaminant material and dispose of it elsewhere.

Phytoremediation consists in mitigating pollutant concentrations in contaminated soils, water, or air, with plants able to contain, degrade, or eliminate metals, pesticides, solvents, explosives, crude oil and its derivatives, and various other contaminants from the media that contain them.

Application

Phytoremediation may be applied wherever the soil or static water environment has become polluted or is suffering ongoing chronic pollution. Examples where phytoremediation has been used successfully include the restoration of abandoned metal-mine workings, reducing the impact of sites where polychlorinated biphenyl have been dumped during manufacture and mitigation of on-going coal mine discharges.

Phytoremediation refers to the natural ability of certain plants called hyperaccumulators to bioaccumulate, degrade,or render harmless contaminants in soils, water,or air. Contaminants such as metals, pesticides, solvents, explosives, and crude oil and its derivatives, have been mitigated in phytoremediation projects worldwide. Many plants such as mustard plants, alpine pennycress, and pigweed have proven to be successful at hyperaccumulating contaminants at toxic-waste sites.

Phytoremediation is considered a clean, cost-effective and non-environmentally disruptive technology, as opposed to mechanical cleanup methods such as soil excavation or pumping polluted groundwater. Over the past 20 years, this technology has become increasingly popular and has been employed at sites with soils contaminated with lead, uranium, and arsenic. However, one major disadvantage of phytoremediation is that it requires a long-term commitment, as the process is dependent on plant growth, tolerance to toxicity, and bioaccumulation capacity.

Phytostabilization

Phytostabilization focuses on long-term stabilization and containment of the pollutant. For example, the plant's presence can reduce wind erosion; or the plant's roots can prevent water erosion, immobilize the pollutants by adsorption or accumulation, and provide a zone around the roots where the pollutant can precipitate and stabilize. Unlike phytoextraction, phytostabilization focuses mainly on sequestering pollutants in soil near the roots but not in plant tissues. Pollutants become less bioavailable, and livestock, wildlife, and human exposure is reduced. An example application of this sort is using a vegetative cap to stabilize and contain mine tailings.

Phytotransformation

In the case of organic pollutants, such as pesticides, explosives, solvents, industrial chemicals, and other xenobiotic substances, certain plants, such as Cannas, render these substances non-toxic by their metabolism. In other cases, microorganisms living in association with plant roots may metabolize these substances in soil or water. These complex and recalcitrant compounds cannot be broken down to basic molecules (water, carbon-dioxide, etc.) by plant molecules, and, hence, the term *phytotransformation* represents a change in chemical structure without complete breakdown of the compound. The term "Green Liver Model" is used to describe phytotransformation, as plants behave analogously to the human liver when dealing with these xenobiotic compounds (foreign compound/pollutant). After uptake of the xenobiotics, plant enzymes increase the polarity of the xenobiotics by adding functional groups such as hydroxyl groups (-OH).

This is known as Phase I metabolism, similar to the way that the human liver increases the polarity of drugs and foreign compounds (Drug Metabolism). Whereas in the human liver enzymes such as Cytochrome P450s are responsible for the initial reactions, in plants enzymes such as nitroreductases carry out the same role.

In the second stage of phytotransformation, known as Phase II metabolism, plant biomolecules such as glucose and amino acids are added to the polarized xenobiotic to further increase the polarity (known as conjugation). This is again similar to the processes occurring in the human pancreas where glucuronidation (addition of glucose molecules by the UGT (e.g. UGT1A1) class of enzymes) and glutathione addition reactions occur on reactive centres of the xenobiotic.

Phase I and II reactions serve to increase the polarity and reduce the toxicity of the compounds, although many exceptions to the rule are seen. The increased polarity also allows for easy transport of the xenobiotic along aqueous channels. In the final stage of phytotransformation (Phase III metabolism), a sequestration of the xenobiotic occurs within the plant. The xenobiotics polymerize in a lignin-like manner and develop a complex structure that is sequestered in the plant. This ensures that the xenobiotic is safely stored, and does not affect the functioning of the plant. However, preliminary studies have shown that these plants can be toxic to small animals (such as snails), and, hence, plants involved in phytotransformation may need to be maintained in a closed enclosure. Hence, the plants reduce toxicity (with exceptions) and sequester the xenobiotics in phytotransformation. Trinitrotoluene phytotransformation has been extensively researched and a transformation pathway has been proposed.

The Role of Genetics

Breeding programs and genetic engineering are powerful methods for enhancing natural phytoremediation capabilities, or for introducing new capabilities into plants. Genes for phytoremediation may originate from a micro-organism or may be transferred from one plant to another variety better adapted to the environmental conditions at the cleanup site. For example, genes encoding a nitroreductase from a bacterium were inserted into tobacco and showed faster removal of TNT and enhanced resistance to the toxic effects of TNT. Researchers have also discovered a mechanism in plants that allows them to grow even when the pollution concentration in the soil is lethal for non-treated plants. Some natural, biodegradable compounds, such as exogenous polyamines, allow the plants to tolerate concentrations of pollutants 500 times higher than untreated plants, and to absorb more pollutants.

Hyperaccumulators and Biotic Interactions

A plant is said to be a hyperaccumulator if it can concentrate the pollutants in a minimum percentage which varies according to the pollutant involved (for example: more than 1000 mg/kg of dry weight for nickel, copper, cobalt, chromium or lead; or more than 10,000 mg/kg for zinc or manganese). This capacity for accumulation is due to hypertolerance, or *phytotolerance*: the result of adaptative evolution from the plants to hostile environments through many generations. A number of interactions may be affected by metal hyperaccumulation, including protection, interferences with neighbour plants of different species, mutualism (including mycorrhizae, pollen and seed dispersal), commensalism, and biofilm.

Phytotreatment

Phytotreatment is an environmental term referring to the cultivation of specialized plants that absorb specific contaminants from the soil through their roots or foliage. This reduces the concentration of contaminants in the soil, but incorporates them into biomasses that may be released back into the environment when the plant dies or is harvested.

Chapter

8

Ecology of Marine Microbial Biofilms

Microbes such as bacteria tend to live in complex colonies called biofilms, where there can resist antibiotics and cause more problems for the immune system. Biofilms comprising millions of bacteria are at the root of many serious chronic infectious diseases such as cystic fibrosis and periodontal disease, as well as industrial contamination, biofouling and biocorrosion.

Yet biofilms also have equal potential for good behaviour, in particular as agents of self-purification in streams and rivers, waste and pollution treatment, or generation of carbon-neutral electricity. These critical properties are derived from the existence of the protective slimy matrix within which members of the community live, preventing attack from both the immune system and antibiotics, but at the same time shielding them from toxic contaminants while breaking down waste or effluent.

The study of biofilms has emerged over the last three decades in various disciplines such as biotechnology, bioengineering or infectious disease research, leading to rapid progress, but also fragmentation and duplication of effort. The European Science Foundation (ESF) has stepped in to unite Europe's effort and bring together scientists with the required skills in relevant fields such as genetics, molecular biology, microscopy, medical microbiology, environmental science and ecology.

As the ESF Biofilm workshop's convenor Tom J. Battin, from the University of Vienna, pointed out, biofilms are involved in most chronic infections, including killers such as cystic fibrosis, and endocarditis in the heart. In cystic fibrosis, excess mucus production in the airways gives sanctuary to bacteria such as Pseudomonas aeruginosa, which actually mop up the dead carcasses of white blood cells sent by the immune system, enabling them to construct their protective biofilm coat.

In this case the immune system is the architect of its own problems, helping create the shield used to repel its own agents, as well as resisting antibiotics. Indeed resistance against antibiotics is itself one of the biggest problems of all associated with biofilms, Battin noted.

"This becomes particularly dramatic for endocarditis patients, as was outlined at the workshop by Annette Moter from the Charite in Berlin," said Battin. Endocarditis is a rare but serious disease in which one of the four heart valves, the heart lining, or heart muscle, are infected by a bacterial biofilm, often comprising streptococci, and become inflamed. As the biofilms are resistant to antibiotics and the immune system's white blood cells, very often the only remedy is surgery, to replace a damaged valve, which can itself cause problems. The hope is that greater understanding will yield new drugs that reach the infected heart valve and break up the biofilm.

As Battin pointed out, biofilms can pose a big problem in large-scale water treatment plants, and yet for the very same reasons can play a positive role in the very same process, breaking down contaminants in waste and natural waters, for example. Further research will help ensure that the positive role is accentuated, while avoiding the problems.

Yet there is also great excitement about an emerging application that could have some potential for green energy production - the use of biofilms to power microbial fuel cells whose fuel could be wastewater, as outlined at the ESF workshop by Cristian Picioreanu, Delft University of Technology. This exploits the ability of bacteria to transfer electrons to metals, which can be the cathode of a fuel cell, via the minute tentacles called phili extending from their surface.

A biofilm is an aggregate of microorganisms in which cells adhere to each other and/or to a surface. These adherent cells are frequently embedded within a self-produced matrix of extracellular polymeric substance (EPS). Biofilm EPS, which is also referred to as *slime* (although not everything described as slime is a biofilm), is a polymeric conglomeration generally composed of extracellular DNA, proteins, and polysaccharides in various configurations. Biofilms may form on living or non-living surfaces, and represent a prevalent mode of microbial life in natural, industrial and hospital settings. The microbial cells growing in a biofilm are physiologically distinct from planktonic cells of the same organism, which, by contrast, are single-cells that may float or swim in a liquid medium.

Microbes form a biofilm in response to many factors, which may include cellular recognition of specific or non-specific attachment sites on a surface, nutritional cues, or in some cases, by exposure of planktonic cells to sub-inhibitory concentrations of antibiotics. When a cell switches to the biofilm mode of growth, it undergoes a phenotypic shift in behaviour in which large suites of genes are differentially regulated.

Formation

Formation of a biofilm begins with the attachment of free-floating microorganisms to a surface. These first colonists adhere to the surface initially through weak, reversible adhesion via van der Waals forces. If the colonists are not immediately separated from the surface, they can anchor themselves more permanently using cell adhesion structures such as pili. The first colonists facilitate the arrival of other cells by providing more diverse adhesion sites and beginning to build the matrix that holds the biofilm together.

Some species are not able to attach to a surface on their own but are often able to anchor themselves to the matrix or directly to earlier colonists. It is during this colonization that the cells are able to communicate via quorum sensing using such products as AHL.

Once colonization has begun, the biofilm grows through a combination of cell division and recruitment. The final stage of biofilm formation is known as development, and is the stage in which the biofilm is established and may only change in shape and size. The development of a biofilm may allow for an aggregate cell colony (or colonies) to be increasingly antibiotic resistant.

Development

There are five stages of biofilm development:

1. Initial attachment
2. Irreversible attachment
3. Maturation I

4. Maturation II
5. Dispersion.

Dispersal

Dispersal of cells from the biofilm colony is an essential stage of the biofilm lifecycle. Dispersal enables biofilms to spread and colonize new surfaces. Enzymes that degrade the biofilm extracellular matrix, such as dispersin B and deoxyribonuclease, may play a role in biofilm dispersal. Biofilm matrix degrading enzymes may be useful as anti-biofilm agents.

Recent evidence has shown that a fatty acid messenger, cis-2-decenoic acid, is capable of inducing dispersion and inhibiting growth of biofilm colonies. Secreted by *Pseudomonas aeruginosa*, this compound induces dispersion in several species of bacteria and the yeast *Candida albicans*.

Properties

Biofilms are usually found on solid substrates submerged in or exposed to an aqueous solution, although they can form as floating mats on liquid surfaces and also on the surface of leaves, particularly in high humidity climates.

Given sufficient resources for growth, a biofilm will quickly grow to be macroscopic. Biofilms can contain many different types of microorganism, e.g. bacteria, archaea, protozoa, fungi and algae; each group performing specialized metabolic functions. However, some organisms will form monospecies films under certain conditions.

Extracellular Matrix

The biofilm is held together and protected by a matrix of excreted polymeric compounds called EPS. EPS is an abbreviation for either extracellular polymeric substance or exopolysaccharide. This matrix protects the cells within it and facilitates communication among them through biochemical signals. Some biofilms have been found to contain water channels that help distribute nutrients and signalling molecules. This matrix is strong enough that under certain conditions, biofilms can become fossilized.

Bacteria living in a biofilm usually have significantly different properties from free-floating bacteria of the same species, as the dense and protected environment of the film allows them to cooperate and interact in various ways. One benefit of this environment is increased resistance to detergents and antibiotics, as the dense extracellular matrix and the outer layer of cells protect the interior of the community. In some cases antibiotic resistance can be increased a thousandfold. Lateral gene transfer is greatly facilitated in biofilms and leads to a more stable biofilm structure.

The concept that biofilms are more resistant to antimicrobials is not completely accurate. For instance the biofilm form of *Pseudomonas aeruginosa* has no greater resistance to antimicrobials, when compared to stationary phase planktonic cells, although, when the biofilm is compared to logarithmic phase planktonic cells, the biofilm does have greater resistance to antimicrobials. This resistance to antibiotics in both stationary phase cells and biofilms may be due to the presence of persister cells.

Examples

Biofilms are ubiquitous. Nearly every species of microorganism, not only bacteria and archaea, have mechanisms by which they can adhere to surfaces and to each other. Biofilms will form on virtually every non-shedding surface in a non-sterile aqueous environment.

- Biofilms can be found on rocks and pebbles at the bottom of most streams or rivers and often form on the surface of stagnant pools of water. In fact, biofilms are important components of food chains in rivers and streams and are grazed by the aquatic invertebrates upon which many fish feed.
- Biofilms can grow in the most extreme environments: from, for example, the extremely hot, briny waters of hot springs ranging from very acidic to very alkaline, to frozen glaciers.
- In the human environment, biofilms can grow in showers very easily since they provide a moist and warm environment for the biofilm to thrive. Biofilms can form inside water and sewage pipes and cause clogging and corrosion. Biofilms on floors and counters can make sanitation difficult in food preparation areas.
- Biofilms in cooling- or heating-water systems are known to reduce heat transfer.
- Biofilms in marine engineering systems, such as pipelines of the offshore oil and gas industry, can lead to substantial corrosion problems. Corrosion is mainly due to abiotic factors; however, at least 20% is caused by microorganisms that are attached to the metal subsurface (i.e., microbially-influenced corrosion).

- Bacterial adhesion to boat hulls serves as the foundation for biofouling of seagoing vessels. Once a film of bacteria forms, it is easier for other marine organisms such as barnacles to attach. Such fouling can reduce maximum vessel speed by up to 20%, prolonging voyages and consuming fuel. Time in dry dock for refitting and repainting reduces the productivity of shipping assets, and the useful life of ships is also reduced due to corrosion and mechanical removal (scraping) of marine organisms from ships' hulls.
- Biofilms can also be harnessed for constructive purposes. For example, many sewage treatment plants include a treatment stage in which waste water passes over biofilms grown on filters, which extract and digest organic compounds. In such biofilms, bacteria are mainly responsible for removal of organic matter (BOD), while protozoa and rotifers are mainly responsible for removal of suspended solids (SS), including pathogens and other microorganisms. Slow sand filters rely on biofilm development in the same way to filter surface water from lake, spring or river sources for drinking purposes. What we regard as clean water is a waste material to these microcellular organisms since they are unable to extract any further nutrition from the purified water.
- Biofilms can help eliminate petroleum oil from contaminated oceans or marine systems. The oil is eliminated by the hydrocarbon-degrading activities of microbial communities, in particular by a remarkable recently-discovered group of specialists, the so-called hydrocarbonoclastic bacteria (HCB).
- Stromatolites are layered accretionary structures formed in shallow water by the trapping, binding and cementation of sedimentary grains by microbial biofilms, especially of cyanobacteria. Stromatolites include some of the most ancient records of life on Earth, and are still forming today.
- Biofilms are present on the teeth of most animals as dental plaque, where they may cause tooth decay and gum disease.
- Biofilms are found on the surface of and inside plants. They can either contribute to crop disease or, as in the case of nitrogen-fixing Rhizobium on roots, exist symbiotically with the plant. Examples of crop diseases related to biofilms include Citrus Canker, Pierce's Disease of grapes, and Bacterial Spot of plants such as peppers and tomatoes.

Biofilms and Infectious Diseases

Biofilms have been found to be involved in a wide variety of microbial infections in the body, by one estimate 80% of all infections. Infectious processes in which biofilms have been implicated include common problems such as urinary tract infections, catheter infections, middle-ear infections, formation of dental plaque, gingivitis, coating contact lenses, and less common but more lethal processes such as endocarditis, infections in cystic fibrosis, and infections of permanent indwelling devices such as joint prostheses and heart valves.

More recently it has been noted that bacterial biofilms may impair cutaneous wound healing and reduce topical antibacterial efficiency in healing or treating infected skin wounds. It has recently been shown that biofilms are present on the removed tissue of 80% of patients undergoing surgery for chronic sinusitis.

The patients with biofilms were shown to have been denuded of cilia and goblet cells, unlike the controls without biofilms who had normal cilia and goblet cell morphology. Biofilms were also found on samples from two of 10 healthy controls mentioned. The species of bacteria from interoperative cultures did not correspond to the bacteria species in the biofilm on the respective patient's tissue.

In other words, the cultures were negative though the bacteria were present. Biofilms can also be formed on the inert surfaces of implanted devices such as catheters, prosthetic cardiac valves and intrauterine devices. New staining techniques are being developed to differentiate bacterial cells growing in living animals, e.g. from tissues with allergy-inflammations .

Pseudomonas Aeruginosa Biofilms

The achievements of medical care in industrialised societies are markedly impaired due to chronic opportunistic infections that have become increasingly apparent in immunocompromised patients and the aging population. Chronic infections remain a major challenge for the medical profession and are of great economic relevance because traditional antibiotic therapy is usually not sufficient to eradicate these infections.

One major reason for persistence seems to be the capability of the bacteria to grow within biofilms that protects them from adverse environmental factors. *Pseudomonas aeruginosa* is not only an important opportunistic pathogen and causative agent of emerging nosocomial infections but can also be considered a model organism for the study of diverse bacterial mechanisms that contribute to bacterial persistence. In this context the elucidation of the molecular mechanisms responsible for the switch from planktonic growth to a biofilm phenotype and the role of inter-bacterial communication in persistent disease should provide new insights in *P. aeruginosa* pathogenicity, contribute to a better clinical management of chronically infected patients and should lead to the identification of new drug targets for the development of alternative anti-infective treatment strategies.

Dental Plaque

Dental plaque is the material that adheres to the teeth and consists of bacterial cells (mainly *Streptococcus mutans* and *Streptococcus sanguinis*), salivary polymers and bacterial extracellular products. Plaque is a biofilm on the surfaces of the teeth. This accumulation of microorganisms subject the teeth and gingival tissues to high concentrations of bacterial metabolites which results in dental disease.

Legionellosis

Legionella bacteria are known to grow under certain conditions in biofilms, in which they are protected against disinfectants. Workers in cooling towers, persons working in air conditioned rooms and people taking a shower are exposed to Legionella by inhalation when the systems are not well designed, constructed, or maintained.

Neisseria Gonorrhoeae Biofilms

Neisseria gonorrhoeae is an exclusive human pathogen. Recent studies have demonstrated that it utilizes two distinct mechanisms for entry into human urethral and cervical epithelial cells involving different bacterial surface ligands and host receptors. In addition it has been demonstrated that the gonococcus can form biofilms on glass surfaces and over human cells. There is evidence for formation of gonococcal biofilms on human cervical epithelial cells during natural disease and that outer membrane blebbing by the gonococcus is crucial in biofilm formation over human cervical epithelial cells.

Molecular Genetics

Technological progress in microscopy, molecular genetics and genome analysis has significantly advanced our understanding of the structural and molecular aspects of biofilms, especially of extensively studied model organisms such as *Pseudomonas aeruginosa*. Biofilm development can be divided into several key steps including attachment, microcolony formation, biofilm maturation and dispersion; and in each step bacteria may recruit different components and molecules including flagellae, type IV pili, DNA and exopolysaccharides.

The rapid progress in biofilm research has also unveiled several genetic regulation mechanisms implicated in biofilm regulation such as quorum sensing and the novel secondary messenger cyclic-di-GMP. Understanding the molecular mechanisms of biofilm formation has facilitated the exploration of novel strategies to control bacterial biofilms.

Screening of Biofouling Activity in Marine Bacterial Isolate from Ship Hull

In the marine environment, competition for living space is intense; therefore, all surfaces living or innate are susceptible to fouling. This process generally begins with the formation of a biochemical conditioning film on to which bacteria and other microorganisms colonize (Costerton and Lappin-Scott, 1995). Closely following the microbial fouling is the colonization of various eukaryotic organisms, including marine invertebrates and algae (Loeb and Neihof, 1975).

Biofouling is divided into microfouling, a biofilm formation and bacterial adhesion and macrofouling, an attachment of larger organisms, of which the culprits are barnacles, mussels, polychaete worms, bryozoans and sea weeds (Melo and Bott, 1997). Biofouling is directly related to the presence of microorganisms which can damage the metal by adhering to different surfaces. Bacterial cells can encase themselves in a hydrated matrix of polysaccharides and proteins and form a slimy layer known as biofilms (Augustin and Vehmas, 2004; Vrouwenvelder *et al.*, 2008). However, surface related attachment does not mean static; biofilms are very dynamic systems.

Their formation is a progressive process in which colonizing bacteria move to or are transported to a surface, attach and through a series of steps, produce a biofilm. The primary colonizers of any fresh surface are predominantly bacteria and diatoms. Marine organisms like *Vibrio proteolyticus* (Paul and Jeffrey, 1985), *Escherichia coli*, *Pseudomonas aeruginosa*, *Shewanella oneidensis* and *Bacillus subtilis* (Omoike and Chorover, 2004) have been found to be involved in the biofouling process. Bacterial colonization occurs via a two step process beginning with reversible attachment to the substratum followed by irreversible adhesion (Dexter, 1979; Morisaki *et al.*, 1999). The reversible attachments of cells are held by physical forces and can be easily removed by gentle washing.

Non reversible attachment of cells is often mediated via specific mechanisms such as hydrogen bonding, cation bridging, specific receptor ligand interactions and the production of extracellular polysaccharides (EPS) (Biancitto *et al.*, 2001; Jayaraman and Seetharaman, 2003). In ships, the adverse effects caused by this biological settlement are high fractional resistance, due to generated roughness, which leads to an increase of weight and subsequent potential speed reduction (Yebra *et al.*, 2004). The biofouling bacteria were collected on October 2007 from biofilm samples at the Royapuram Harbour, Chennai, Tamil Nadu, India and screened for the biofouling activity.

Materials and Methods

Sample Collection

The biofilm samples were scraped from three different ships anchored at the Royapuram Harbour, Chennai, Tamil Nadu and were brought to the laboratory in sterile polythene bags for further investigation.

Isolation of Bacteria

The collected samples were serially diluted and plated over Zobell agar plates. The inoculated plates were incubated at 28 ± 2 °C for 24-48 h. After incubation, the selected bacterial colonies were purified and subcultured in nutrient agar medium for further investigation (Saravanan *et al.*, 2008).

Screening of Biofouling Activity in Bacterial Isolates by Microtiter Plate Assay

The bacterial isolates were grown over night in nutrient broth at 37 °C. Aliquots of 3 ìL were inoculated in six parallel wells of a 96 well microtiter plate. Then the plate was incubated at 37 °C for 72 h. After the incubation period, the wells were rinsed with physiological saline to remove the detached cells and fixed with 2 ìL of 99.99 % ethanol for 10 min.

The attached bacterial material was then stained adding 2 ìL of crystal violet (2 %) for 20 min. The plate was rinsed with tap water and the amounts of attached cells were measured using an ELISA reader at 570 nm.

Characterization of Biofouling Bacteria Morphological and Biochemical Characterization

The isolate which showed maximum biofouling activity was then characterized using various morphological, biochemical and molecular characters. Gram staining and motility tests were performed for preliminary identification of the isolate (Allegrucci and Sauer, 2007). Morphological parameters include colony color, size, shape and margin; biochemical tests such as catalase, sugar fermentation and nitrate reduction were carried out (Dalton *et al.*, 1994).

Molecular Characterization

The chromosomal DNA was isolated (Bollet *et al.*, 1955) from the DR4 isolate by alkali lysis method and subsequently amplified by PCR using the universal forward and reverse primers 5' AGAGTTTGATC CTGGCTCAG3' and 5'ACGGCTACC-TTGTTACG ACT3', respectively.

The following parameters were used for PCR (Weisburg *et al.*, 1991) amplification: 30 cycles of initial denaturation step at 94 °C for 2 min, followed by denaturation step at 94 °C for 45 sec, annealing at 52 °C for 30 sec, extension at 72 °C for 1 min and final extension at 72 °C for 2 min. The PCR product was resolved by 1 % agarose gel stained with ethidium bromide and the amplicon was sent for sequencing to First-Base, Singapore. Specific primer 5'GTATTACCGCGGCGTGCTGG 3' was provided along with the sample for sequencing.

The nucleotide sequence obtained was compared with the known bacterial sequences available in the NCBI database using the bioinformatics tool BLAST and a phylogenetic tree was constructed using the PHYLIP program (Janet *et al.*, 2000). The secondary structure of the bacterial 16S rDNA was predicted using Genbee software. The restriction sites present on the bacterial 16S rDNA was analyzed using the NEB Cutter program.

Results and Discussion

In the present study, the biofilm samples were collected from three different ships. The samples were plated on Zobell agar medium for bacterial isolation. Totally 11 isolates were obtained: 3 isolates from ship I, 3 isolates from ship II and 5 isolates from ship III.

The diversity of bacterial isolate was increased due to the nutritive status of water. The biofouling bacteria have already been reported from different habitats. Sillankorva *et al.* (2008) has isolated *Pseudomonas fluorescence* from biofilm samples, Kreig and Hoit (1984) and Sonak and Bhosle (1995) have isolated *Vibrio alginolyticus* from Tin panel associated biofilm, Chaudhary *et al.* (1996) have isolated *Aerobacter aerogens* and *Bacillus alvei* from various sites within a paper mill and Nidal *et al.* (2004) have isolated *Escherichia coli* from membrane systems.

Thus, it is obvious that *Bacillus* spp. is adapted to diverse habitats which vary widely in space and time and also diverse environmental conditions. Totally 11 isolates were obtained from three ships and named as RB1, RB1a, RB1b, RB2, RB21, RB22, DR1, DR2, DR3, DR4 and DR5. Among the 11 isolates, only DR4 showed maximum biofouling activity in the microtitre plate assay with a significant optical density (OD) of 0.596.

The other isolates did not show significant biofouling activity.The microtitre plate method was done by Abdi-Ali *et al.* (2006). A similar biofilm screening has been done by Bhosale *et al.* (2002) using floating glass cover slips on the sterilized filtered sea water to check the adherence of *Bacillus* spp. and *Pseudomonas* spp., biofilms and then staining the cover slips with gentian violet. The different parameters namely morphological, biochemical and molecular characters were used for characterization and identification of bacterial isolate. The bacterial isolate DR4 was observed as pale colored circular colonies on Zobell agar medium. The staining report showed gram positive, rod shaped and nonmotile cells. Various biochemical characteristics of biofouling bacteria were used for their identification.

In the present investigation, it was found that the bacterial isolate DR4 was found to be positive for catalase. It can ferment glucose, maltose and sucrose and reduced nitrates to nitrites. Rajasekar *et al.* (2007) reported the presence of *Bacillus* spp., in corrosion product of pipe line and were characterized depending upon morphology, gram staining and biochemical tests. The classification of bacteria using morphological and physiological characteristics does not necessarily lead to the identification of phylogenetically coherent taxa.

However, some of these characters were shown to be variable with changing media and environmental conditions. Several chemotaxonomic markers (isozyme patterns, fatty acid profile etc.) were used for species and strain level differentiation with little success. To evaluate the bacteria, different polymerase chain reaction (PCR) based molecular methods namely 16S rDNA sequencing, randomly amplified polymorphic DNA (RAPD), short tandemly repeated repetitive (STRR), etc. may be used at all taxonomic levels. The sequence analysis of genes encoding 16S rDNA is currently the most promising approach for phylogenetic classification of bacteria. The comparison of rDNA sequence is a powerful tool for detecting phylogenetic and evolutionary relationship among bacterial species.

In the present study, the DNA was isolated from the bacterial isolate DR4 and was analyzed by agarose gel electrophoresis. A sharp band of genomic DNA was obtained in the gel and 50 ng of DNA was used as template. The amplification 16S rDNA gene of the bacterial isolate DR4 was performed by PCR technique using universal primers. A sharp band was observed in 1 % agarose gel which confirmed the presence of 16S rDNA. The amplified 16S rDNA sample was sent to First-Base, Singapore for sequencing. The obtained nucleotide 16S rDNA sequence for the bacterial isolate DR4 was used for the basic local alignment search tool (BLAST) and the sequence showed similarity with the *Bacillus* sp. A phylogenetic tree of the isolate DR4 was constructed using its 16S rDNA sequence with that of the other *Bacillus* sp. obtained from the NCBI database. The resultant phylogenetic tree showed similarity of the isolate DR4 only at the genus level, whereas it did not show any similarity at the species level, hence DR4 was found in a separate branch. A similar kind of results has been reported for *Bacillus subtilis* strains isolated from the biofilms of Gulf of Mexico (Jenet *et al.*, 2000). The secondary structure of the bacterial 16S rDNA was showed 27 loops and 36 stems with an overall free energy of -190.1 kkal/mol. The restriction sites present on the bacterial 16S rDNA showed 55 restriction sites and 42 % and 58 % GC and AC contents, respectively.

The present study gives an idea about the presence of biofouling bacteria *Bacillus* sp., in the marine biofilm samples. It was characterized and identified using different parameters such as morphological, biochemical and molecular characters. Identifying a suitable natural antifouling agent against this biofouling bacterium is thus suggested as further course of action.

Conclusion

The present investigation has clearly revealed the presence of biofouling bacteria in the marine biofilm samples collected from the ships anchored in the Royapuram harbour, Chennai, India. Morphological, biochemical and molecular characterization studies showed the diversity of different strains of *Bacillus* spp. and the biofouling activity of *Bacillus* sp. DR4. In order to minimize the economic loss, fuel consumption and metal corrosion due to the formation of biofilms, there is an urgent need for identifying suitable natural antifouling agents to control the biofouling bacteria which is abundant in the marine environments.

Environmental Biosphere

The biosphere is the region of the earth that encompasses all living organisms: plants, animals and bacteria. It is a feature that distinguishes the earth from the other planets in the solar system. "Bio" means life, and the term biosphere was first coined by a Russian scientist (Vladimir Vernadsky) in the 1920s. Another term sometimes used is ecosphere ("eco" meaning home). The biosphere includes the outer region of the earth (the lithosphere) and the lower region of the atmosphere (the troposphere).

It also includes the hydrosphere, the region of lakes, oceans, streams, ice and clouds comprising the earth's water resources. Traditionally, the biosphere is considered to extend from the bottom of the oceans to the highest mountaintops, a layer with an average thickness of about 20 kilometers. Scientists now know that some forms of microbes live at great depths, sometimes several thousand meters into the earth's crust. Nonetheless, the biosphere is a very tiny region on the scale of the whole earth, analogous to the thickness of the skin on an apple. The bulk of living organisms actually live within a smaller fraction of the biosphere, from about 500 meters below the ocean's surface to about 6 kilometers above sea level.

Dynamic interactions occur between the biotic region (biosphere) and the abiotic regions (atmosphere, lithosphere and hydrosphere) of the earth. Energy, water, gases and nutrients are exchanged between the regions on various spatial and time scales. Such exchanges depend upon, and can be altered by, the environments of the regions. For example, the chemical processes of early life on earth (e.g. photosynthesis, respiration, carbonate formation) transformed the reducing ancient atmosphere into the oxidizing (free oxygen) environment of today. The interactive processes between the biosphere and the abiotic regions work to maintain a kind of planetary equilibrium. These processes, as well as those that might disrupt this equilibrium, involve a range of scientific and socioeconomic issues.

The study of the relationships of living organisms with one another and with their environment is the science known as ecology. The word ecology comes from the Greek words oikos and logos, and literally means "study of the home." The ecology of the earth can be studied at various levels: an individual (organism), a population, a community, an ecosystem, a biome or the entire biosphere. The variety of living organisms that inhabit an environment is a measure of its biodiversity.

Organisms

Life evolved after oceans formed, as the ocean environment provided the necessary nutrients and support medium for the initial simple organisms. It also protected them from the harsh atmospheric UV radiation. As organisms became more complex they eventually became capable of living on land. However, this could not occur until the atmosphere became oxidizing and a protective ozone layer formed which blocked the harmful UV radiation. Over roughly the last four billion years, organisms have diversified and adapted to all kinds of environments, from the icy regions near the poles to the warm tropics near the equator, and from deep in the rocky crust of the earth to the upper reaches of the troposphere. Despite their diversity, all living organisms share certain characteristics: they all replicate and all use DNA to accomplish the replication process. Based on the structure of their cells, organisms can be classified into two types: eukaryotes and prokaryotes.

The main difference between them is that a eukaryote has a nucleus, which contains its DNA, while a prokaryote does not have a nucleus, but instead its DNA is free-floating in the cell. Bacteria are prokaryotes, and humans are eukaryotes. Organisms can also be classified according to how they acquire energy. Autotrophs are "self feeders" that use light or chemical energy to make food. Plants are autotrophs. Heterotrophs (i.e. other feeders) obtain energy by eating other organisms, or their remains. Bacteria and animals are heterotrophs. Groups of organisms that are physically and genetically related can be classified into species. There are millions of species on the earth, most of them unstudied and many of them unknown. Insects and microorganisms comprise the majority of species, while humans and other mammals comprise only a tiny fraction. In an ecological study, a single member of a species or organism is known as an individual.

Populations and Communities

A number of individuals of the same species in a given area constitute a population. The number typically ranges anywhere from a few individuals to several thousand individuals. Bacterial populations can number in the millions. Populations live in a place or environment called a habitat. All of the populations of species in a given region together make up a community. In an area of tropical grassland, a community might be made up of grasses, shrubs, insects, rodents and various species of hoofed mammals. The populations and communities found in a particular environment are determined by abiotic and biotic limiting factors. These are the factors that most affect the success of populations. Abiotic limiting factors involve the physical and chemical characteristics of the environment. Some of these factors include: amounts of sunlight, annual rainfall, available nutrients, oxygen levels and temperature.

For example, the amount of annual rainfall may determine whether a region is a grassland or forest, which in turn, affects the types of animals living there. Each population in a community has a range of tolerance for an abiotic limiting factor. There are also certain maximum and minimum requirements known as tolerance limits, above and below which no member of a population is able to survive. The range of an abiotic factor that results in the largest population of a species is known as the optimum range for that factor. Some populations may have a narrow range of tolerance for one factor. For example, a freshwater fish species may have a narrow tolerance range for dissolved oxygen in the water. If the lake in which that fish species lives undergoes eutrophication, the species will die. This fish species can therefore act as an indicator species, because its presence or absence is a strict indicator of the condition of the lake with regard to dissolved oxygen content.

Biotic limiting factors involve interactions between different populations, such as competition for food and habitat. For example, an increase in the population of a meat-eating predator might result in a decrease in the population of its plant-eating prey, which in turn might result in an increase in the plant population the prey feeds on. Sometimes, the presence of a certain species may significantly affect the community make up. Such a species is known as a keystone species. For example, a beaver builds a dam on a stream and causes the meadow behind it to flood. A starfish keeps mussels from dominating a rocky beach, thereby allowing many other species to exist there.

Ecosystems

An ecosystem is a community of living organisms interacting with each other and their environment. Ecosystems occur in all sizes. A tidal pool, a pond, a river, an alpine meadow and an oak forest are all examples of ecosystems. Organisms living in a particular ecosystem are adapted to the prevailing abiotic and biotic conditions. Abiotic conditions involve both physical and chemical factors (e.g., sunlight, water, temperature, soil, prevailing wind, latitude and elevation). In order to understand the flow of energy and matter within an ecosystem, it is necessary to study the feeding relationships of the living organisms within it.

Living organisms in an ecosystem are usually grouped according to how they obtain food. Autotrophs that make their own food are known as producers, while heterotrophs that eat other organisms, living or dead, are known as consumers. The producers include land and aquatic plants, algae and microscopic phytoplankton in the ocean. They all make their own food by using chemicals and energy sources from their environment.

For example, plants use photosynthesis to manufacture sugar (glucose) from carbon dioxide and water. Using this sugar and other nutrients (e.g., nitrogen, phosphorus) assimilated by their roots, plants produce a variety of organic materials. These materials include: starches, lipids, proteins and nucleic acids. Energy from sunlight is thus fixed as food used by themselves and by consumers.

The consumers are classed into different groups depending on the source of their food. Herbivores (e.g. deer, squirrels) feed on plants and are known as primary consumers. Carnivores (e.g. lions, hawks, killer whales) feed on other consumers and can be classified as secondary consumers. They feed on primary consumers. Tertiary consumers feed on other carnivores. Some organisms known as omnivores (e.g., bears, rats and humans) feed on both plants and animals. Organisms that feed on dead organisms are called scavengers (e.g., vultures, ants and flies). Detritivores (detritus feeders, e.g. earthworms, termites, crabs) feed on organic wastes or fragments of dead organisms.

Decomposers (e.g. bacteria, fungi) also feed on organic waste and dead organisms, but they digest the materials outside their bodies. The decomposers play a crucial role in recycling nutrients, as they reduce complex organic matter into inorganic nutrients that can be used by producers. If an organic substance can be broken down by decomposers, it is called biodegradable.

In every ecosystem, each consumer level depends upon lower-level organisms (e.g. a primary consumer depends upon a producer, a secondary consumer depends upon a primary consumer and a tertiary consumer depends upon a secondary consumer). All of these levels, from producer to tertiary consumer, form what is known as a food chain. A community has many food chains that are interwoven into a complex food web. The amount of organic material in a food web is referred to as its biomass.

When one organism eats another, chemical energy stored in biomass is transferred from one level of the food chain to the next. Most of the consumed biomass is not converted into biomass of the consumer. Only a small portion of the useable energy is actually transferred to the next level, typically 10 percent. Each higher level of the food chain represents a cumulative loss of useable energy. The result is a pyramid of energy flow, with producers forming the base level. Assuming 10 percent efficiency at each level, the tertiary consumer level would use only 0.1 percent of the energy available at the initial producer level. Because there is less energy available high on the energy pyramid, there are fewer top-level consumers. A disruption of the producer base of a food chain, therefore, has its greatest effect on the top-level consumer.

Ecosystem populations constantly fluctuate in response to changes in the environment, such as rainfall, mean temperature, and available sunlight. Normally, such changes are not drastic enough to significantly alter ecosystems, but catastrophic events such as floods, fires and volcanoes can devastate communities and ecosystems. It may be long after such a catastrophic event before a new, mature ecosystem can become established. After severe disturbance the make up of a community is changed. The resulting community of species changes, as early, post disturbance, fast-growing species are out-competed by other species. This natural process is called ecological succession. It involves two types of succession: primary succession and secondary succession.

Primary succession is the development of the first biota in a given region where no life is found. An example is of this is the surrounding areas where volcanic lava has completely covered a region or has built up a new island in the ocean. Initially, only pioneer species can survive there, typically lichens and mosses, which are able to withstand poor conditions.

They are able to survive in highly exposed areas with limited water and nutrients. Lichen, which is made up of both a fungus and an alga, survives by mutualism. The fungus produces an acid, which acts to further dissolve the barren rock. The alga uses those exposed nutrients, along with photosynthesis, to produce food for both. Grass seeds may land in the cracks, carried by wind or birds. The grass grows, further cracking the rocks, and upon completing its own life cycle, contributes organic matter to the crumbling rock to make soil. In time, larger plants, such as shrubs and trees may inhabit the area, offering habitats and niches to immigrating animal life. When the maximum biota that the ecosystem can support is reached, the climax community prevails. This occurs after hundreds if not thousands of years depending on the climate and location.

Secondary succession begins at a different point, when an existing ecosystem's community of species is removed by fire, deforestation, or a bulldozer's work in a vacant lot, leaving only soil. The first few centimeters of this soil may have taken 1000 years to develop from solid rock. It may be rich in humus, organic waste, and may be stocked with ready seeds of future plants. Secondary succession is also a new beginning, but one with a much quicker regrowth of organisms. Depending on the environment, succession to a climax community may only require 100 to 200 years with normal climate conditions, with communities progressing through stages of early plant and animal species, mid-species and late successional species. Some ecosystems, however, can never by regained.

The grass grows, further cracking the rocks and upon completing its own life cycle, contributes organic content to the crumbling rock becoming soil. In time, larger plants then shrubs then trees may dominate this area, offering habitats and niches to immigrating animal life. Reaching the maximum biota this ecosystem can support, the climax community caps off further succession after hundreds if not thousands of years depending on the climate and location. Secondary succession begins at a different point. Due to a disturbance to an existing ecosystem, such as fire, deforestation, farmland left abandoned, or even the bulldozer's work in a vacant lot, biota are removed. What does remain, however, is the soil. Soil that may have taken 1000 years to develop the first centimeter from solid rock. Soil that may be rich in humus, organic wastes. Soil that may be stocked with ready seeds of future plants. Secondary succession is also new beginning, but with the advantage of quick regrowth of organisms.

Once underway, the ecosystem's succession to its climax community may only require 100-200 years with normal climate conditions, progressing just like the primary succession through stages of early plant and animal species, mid-species, and late successional species.

Biomes

The biosphere can be divided into relatively large regions called biomes. A biome has a distinct climate and certain living organisms (especially vegetation) characteristic to the region and may contain many ecosystems. The key factors determining climate are average annual precipitation and temperature. These factors, in turn, depend on the geography of the region, such as the latitude and elevation of the region, and mountainous barriers. The major types of biomes include: aquatic, desert, forest, grassland and tundra. Biomes have no distinct boundaries. Instead, there is a transition zone called an ecotone, which contains a variety of plants and animals. For example, an ecotone might be a transition region between a grassland and a desert, with species from both.

Water covers a major portion of the earth's surface, so aquatic biomes contain a rich diversity of plants and animals. Aquatic biomes can be subdivided into two basic types: freshwater and marine. Freshwater has a low salt concentration, usually less than 1 percent, and occurs in several types of regions: ponds and lakes, streams and rivers, and wetlands. Ponds and lakes range in size, and small ponds may be seasonal. They sometimes have limited species diversity due to isolation from other water environments. They can get their water from precipitation, surface runoff, rivers, and springs. Streams and rivers are bodies of flowing water moving in one general direction (i.e., downstream). Streams and rivers start at their upstream headwaters, which could be springs, snowmelt or even lakes.

They continue downstream to their mouths, which may be another stream, river, lake or ocean. The environment of a stream or river may change along its length, ranging from clear, cool water near the head, to warm, sediment-rich water near the mouth. The greatest diversity of living organisms usually occurs in the middle region. Wetlands are places of still water that support aquatic plants, such as cattails, pond lilies and cypress trees. Types of wetlands include marshes, swamps and bogs. Wetlands have the highest diversity of species with many species of birds, fur-bearing mammals, amphibians and reptiles. Some wetlands, such as salt marshes, are not freshwater regions.

Marine regions cover nearly three-fourths of the earth's surface. Marine bodies are salty, having approximately 35 grams of dissolved salt per liter of water (3.5 percent). Oceans are very large marine bodies that dominate the earth's surface and hold the largest ecosystems. They contain a rich diversity of living organisms. Ocean regions can be separated into four major zones: intertidal, pelagic, benthic and abyssal. The intertidal zone is where the ocean meets the land. Sometimes, it is submerged and at other times exposed, depending upon waves and tides. The pelagic zone includes the open ocean further away from land. The benthic zone is the region below the pelagic zone, but not including the very deepest parts of the ocean. The bottom of this zone consists of sediments. The deepest parts of the ocean are known as the abyssal zone. This zone is very cold (near freezing temperatures), and under great pressure from the overlying mass of water. Mid-ocean ridges occur on the ocean floor in abyssal zones. Coral reefs are found in the warm, clear, shallow waters of tropical oceans around islands or along continental coastlines.

They are mostly formed from calcium carbonate produced by living coral. Reefs provide food and shelter for other organisms and protect shorelines from erosion. Estuaries are partially enclosed areas where fresh water and silt from streams or rivers mix with salty ocean water. They represent a transition from land to sea and from freshwater to saltwater. Estuaries are biologically very productive areas and provide homes for a wide variety of plants, birds and animals. Deserts have relatively little vegetation and the substrate consists mostly of sand, gravel or rocks. The transition regions between deserts and grasslands are sometimes called semiarid deserts (e.g. the Great Basin of the western United States).

Grasslands cover regions where moderate rainfall is sufficient for the growth of grasses, but not enough for stands of trees. There are two main types of grasslands: tropical grasslands (savannas) and temperate grasslands. Tropical grasslands occur in warm climates such as Africa and very limited regions of Australia. They have a few scattered trees and shrubs, but their distinct rainy and dry seasons prevent the formation of tropical forests. Lower rainfall, more variable winter-through-summer temperatures and a near lack of trees characterize temperate grasslands. Prairies are temperate grasslands at fairly high elevation. They may be dominated by long or short grass species.

The vast prairies originally covering central North America, or the Great Plains, were the result of favorable climate conditions created by their high elevation and proximity to the Rocky Mountains. Because temperate grasslands are treeless, relatively flat and have rich soil, most have been replaced by farmland.

Forests are dominated by trees and can be divided into three types: tropical forests, temperate forests and boreal forests. Tropical forests are always warm and wet and are found at lower latitudes. Their annual precipitation is very high, although some regions may have distinct wet and dry seasons. Tropical forests have the highest biodiversity of this biome. Temperate forests occur at mid-latitudes (i.e., North America), and therefore have distinct seasons. Summers are warm and winters are cold. The temperate forests have suffered considerable alteration by humans, who have cleared much of the forest land for fuel, building materials and agricultural use. Boreal forests are located in higher latitudes, like Siberia, where they are known as "taiga."

They have very long, cold winters and a short summer season when most of the precipitation occurs. Boreal forests represent the largest biome on the continents.

Very low temperatures, little precipitation and low biodiversity characterize tundra. Its vegetation is very simple, with virtually no trees. The tundra can be divided into two different types: arctic tundra and alpine tundra. The arctic alpine occurs in polar regions. It has a very short summer growing season. Water collects in ponds and bogs, and the ground has a subsurface layer of permanently frozen soil known as permafrost. Alpine tundra is found at high elevations in tall mountains. The temperatures are not as low as in the arctic tundra, and it has a longer summer growing season.

Evolution of Life

Wherever they are found in the biosphere, living organisms are necessarily linked to their environment. Ecosystems are dynamic and communities change over time in response to abiotic or biotic changes in the environment. For example, the climate may be become warmer or colder, wetter or drier, or the food chain may be disrupted by the loss of a particular population or the introduction of a new one. Species must be able to adapt to these changes in order to survive. As they adapt, the organisms themselves undergo change. Evolution is the gradual change in the genetic makeup of a population of a species over time. It is important to note that it is the population that evolves, rather than individuals.

A species evolves to a particular niche either by adapting to use a niche's environment or adapting to avoid competition with another species. Recall that no two species can occupy the exact same niche in an ecosystem. The availability of resources is pivotal.

In the case of five warbler species which all consume insects of the same tree, to survive each species needs to gather its food (insects) in different parts of that tree. This avoids competition and the possible extinction of one or more species. Therefore, one of the bird species will adapt to hunting at the treetops; another the lowest branches; another the mid-section. In this way, these species have evolved into different, yet similar, niches. All five species in this way can survive by adapting to a narrow niche. Organisms with a narrow niche are called specialized species. Another example is a species that may evolve to a narrow niche by consuming only one type of leaf, such as the Giant Panda, which consumes bamboo leaves.

This strategy allows it to co-exist with another consumer by not competing with it. In both cases, species with a narrow niche are often vulnerable to extinction because they typically cannot respond to changes in the environment. Evolving to a new niche would take too much time for the specialized species under the duress of a drought, for example. On the other hand, a species that can use many foods and locations in which to hunt or gather are known as generalized species. In the event of a drought, a generalized species such as a cockroach may be more successful in finding alternative forms of food, and will survive and reproduce.

Yet another form of evolution is co-evolution, where species adapt to one another by interacting closely. This relationship can be a predator-prey type of interaction. Prey is at risk, but as a species it has evolved chemical defenses or behaviours. On the other hand, co-evolution can be a mutualistic relationship, often characterized by the ants and an acacia tree of South America. The acacia provides ants with food and a habitat, and its large projecting thorns provides protection from predators. The ants, in turn, protect the tree by attacking any animal landing on it and by clearing vegetation at its base. So closely evolved are the species that neither can exist without the other. Similar ecosystems may offer similar niches to organisms, that are adapted or evolved to that niche. Convergent evolution is the development of similar adaptations in two species occupying different yet similar ecosystems. Two species evolve independently to respond to the demands of their ecosystem, and they develop the same mechanism to do so. What emerges are adaptations that resemble look-alikes: Wings of birds and bats are similar, but evolved separately to meet the demands of flying through air. The dolphin, a mammal, shares adaptations that allow for movement through water with the extinct reptile ichthyosaur. They have similar streamlined shapes of fins, head, and nose, which make the bodies better suited for swimming. Natural selection is another process that depends on an organism's ability to survive in a changing environment. While evolution is the gradual change of the genetic makeup over time, natural selection is the force that favors a beneficial set of genes.

For example, birds migrating to an island face competition for the insects on a tropical tree. One genetic pool of a new generation may include a longer beak, which allows the bird to reach into a tropical flower for its nectar. When high populations of birds compete for insects, this ability to use the niche of collecting nectar favours that bird's survival. The long-beaked gene is passed to the next generation and the next, because birds can coexist with the insect-gathering birds by using a different niche. Through reproduction of the surviving longer-beaked birds, natural selection favours its adaptability. A species, family or larger group of organisms may eventually come to the end of its evolutionary line. This is known as extinction. While bad news for those that become extinct, it's a natural occurrence that has been taking place since the beginning of life on earth. Extinctions of species are constantly occurring at some background rate, which is normally matched by speciation. Thus, in the natural world, there is a constant turnover of species.

Occasionally large numbers of species have become extinct over a relatively short geologic time period. The largest mass extinction event in the earth's history occurred at the end of the Permian period, 245 million years ago. As many as 96 percent of all marine species were lost, while on land more than 75 percent of all vertebrate families became extinct. Although, the actual cause of that extinction is unclear, the consensus is that climate change, resulting from sea level change and increased volcanic activity, was an important factor. The most famous of all mass extinctions occurred at the boundary of the Cretaceous and Tertiary periods, 65 million years ago. About 85 percent of species became extinct, including all of the dinosaurs. Most scientists believe that the impact of a small asteroid near the Yucatan Peninsula in Mexico triggered that extinction event. The impact probably induced a dramatic change in the world climate. The most serious extinction of mammals occurred about 11,000 years ago, as the last Ice Age was ending. Over a period of just a few centuries, most of the large mammals around the world, such as the mammoth, became extinct. While climate change may have been a factor in their extinction, a new force had also emerged on the earth - modern humans. Humans, aided by new, sharp-pointed weapons and hunting techniques, may have hurried the demise of the large land mammals. Over the years, human activity has continued to send many species to an early extinction. The best known examples are the passenger pigeon and the dodo bird, but numerous other species, many of them unknown, are killed off by over harvesting and other human-caused habitat destruction, degradation and fragmentation.

Our biosphere is the global sum of all ecosystems. It can also be called the zone of life on Earth, a closed (apart from solar and cosmic radiation) and self-regulating system. From the broadest biophysiological point of view, the biosphere is the global ecological system integrating all living beings and their relationships, including their interaction with the elements of the lithosphere, hydrosphere and atmosphere.

The biosphere is postulated to have evolved, beginning through a process of biogenesis or biopoesis, at least some 3.5 billion years ago. In a broader sense; biospheres are any closed, self-regulating systems containing ecosystems; including artificial ones such as Biosphere 2 and BIOS-3; and, potentially, ones on other planets or moons.

Origin and Use of the Term

The term "biosphere" was coined by geologist Eduard Suess in 1875, which he defined as:

"The place on Earth's surface where life dwells."

While this concept has a geological origin, it is an indication of the impact of both Darwin and Maury on the earth sciences. The biosphere's ecological context comes from the 1920s, preceding the 1935 introduction of the term "ecosystem" by Sir Arthur Tansley. Vernadsky defined ecology as the science of the biosphere. It is an interdisciplinary concept for integrating astronomy, geophysics, meteorology, biogeography, evolution, geology, geochemistry, hydrology and, generally speaking, all life and earth sciences.

Gaia Hypothesis

The concept that the biosphere is itself a living organism, either actually or metaphorically, is known as the Gaia hypothesis. James Lovelock, an atmospheric scientist from the United Kingdom, proposed the Gaia hypothesis to explain how biotic and abiotic factors interact in the biosphere. This hypothesis considers Earth itself a kind of living organism. Its atmosphere, geosphere, and hydrosphere are cooperating systems that yield a biosphere full of life. In the early 1970s, Lynn Margulis, a microbiologist from the United States, added to the hypothesis, specifically noting the ties between the biosphere and other Earth systems. For example, when carbon dioxide levels increase in the atmosphere, plants grow more quickly. As their growth continues, they remove more and more carbon dioxide from the atmosphere.

Many scientists are now involved in new fields of study that examine interactions between biotic and abiotic factors in the biosphere, such as geobiology and geomicrobiology.

Ecosystems occur when communities and their physical environment work together as a system. The difference between this and a biosphere is simple, the biosphere is everything in general terms.

Extent of Earth's Biosphere

Every part of the planet, from the polar ice caps to the Equator, supports life of some kind. Recent advances in microbiology have demonstrated that microbes live deep beneath the Earth's terrestrial surface, and that the total mass of microbial life in so-called "uninhabitable zones" may, in biomass, exceed all animal and plant life on the surface. The actual thickness of the biosphere on earth is difficult to measure. Birds typically fly at altitudes of 650 to 1,800 meters, and fish that live deep underwater can be found down to -8,372 meters in the Puerto Rico Trench. There are more extreme examples for life on the planet: Rüppell's Vulture has been found at altitudes of 11,300 meters; Bar-headed Geese migrate at altitudes of at least 8,300 meters (over Mount Everest); Yaks live at elevations between 3,200 to 5,400 meters above sea level; mountain goats live up to 3,050 meters. Herbivorous animals at these elevations depend on lichens, grasses, and herbs.

Microscopic organisms live at such extremes that, taking them into consideration puts the thickness of the biosphere much greater. Culturable microbes have been found in the Earth's upper atmosphere as high as 41 km (25 mi) (Wainwright et al., 2003, in FEMS Microbiology Letters).

It is unlikely, however, that microbes are active at such altitudes, where temperatures and air pressure are extremely low and ultraviolet radiation very high. More likely these microbes were brought into the upper atmosphere by winds or possibly volcanic eruptions. Barophilic marine microbes have been found at more than 10 km (6 mi) depth in the Marianas Trench (Takamia et al., 1997, in FEMS Microbiology Letters).

Microbes are not limited to the air, water or the Earth's surface. Culturable thermophilic microbes have been extracted from cores drilled more than 5 km (3 mi) into the Earth's crust in Sweden (Gold, 1992, and Szewzyk, 1994, both in PNAS), from rocks between 65-75 °C. Temperature increases with increasing depth into the Earth's crust.

The speed at which the temperature increases depends on many factors, including type of crust (continental vs. oceanic), rock type, geographic location, etc. The upper known limit of microbial is 122 °C (*Methanopyrus kandleri* Strain 116), and it is likely that the limit of life in the "deep biosphere" is defined by temperature rather than absolute depth.

Our biosphere is divided into a number of biomes, inhabited by broadly similar flora and fauna. On land, biomes are separated primarily by latitude. Terrestrial biomes lying within the Arctic and Antarctic Circles are relatively barren of plant and animal life, while most of the more populous biomes lie near the equator. Terrestrial organisms in temperate and Arctic biomes have relatively small amounts of total biomass, smaller energy budgets, and display prominent adaptations to cold, including world-spanning migrations, social adaptations, homeothermy, estivation and multiple layers of insulation.

Specific Biospheres

When the word is followed by a number, it is usually referring to a specific system or number. Thus:

- Biosphere 1, the planet Earth
- Biosphere 2, a laboratory in Arizona which contains 3.15 acres (13,000 m^2) of closed ecosystem.
- BIOS-3, a closed ecosystem at the Institute of Biophysics in Krasnoyarsk, Siberia, in what was then the Soviet Union.
- Biosphere J (CEEF, Closed Ecology Experiment Facilities), an experiment in Japan.

Chapter

9

Environmental Microbiology of Waste-water Treatment

Microorganisms are significant in water and wastewater because of their roles in different transmission and they are the primary agents of biological treatment.

They are the most divers group of living organisms on earth and occupy important place in the ecosystem. Are called Ommnipresent.

Classification of Bacteria

Classification of Bacteria based on Oxygen Requirements (ORP)

The heterotrophic bacteria are grouped into three classification, depending on their action toward free oxygen (O_4) or more precisely oxygen-reduction potential (ORP) for survival and optimum growth.

1. Obligate aerobe or Aerobes or bacteria are micro-organisms require free dissolved oxygen to oxidize organic mate and to live and multiply. These conditions are referred to as aerobic processes.
2. Anaerobes or anaerobic bacteria are micro-organisms oxidize organic matter in the complete absence of dissolved oxygen. The micro-organisms take oxygen from inorganic sates which contain bound oxygen (Nitrate NO_3, Sulphate So_4^{2-}, Phosphate PO_4^{2-}). This mode of operation is termed as anaerobic process.

3. Facultative bacteria are a class of batter that use free dissolved oxygen when available but can also.

Respire and multiply in the absence. "Escherichia Coli" a facile coli from is a facultative elaterium. (Facultative Bacteria = Aerobic anaerobic bacteria).

Classification of Microorganisms by Kingdom

Microorganisms are organized into five broad groups based on their structural functional differences. The groups are called "Kingdoms". The five kingdoms are animals, plants, protista fungi and bacteria.

Classification by their Preferred Temperature Regimes

Each specie of bacteria reproduces best within a limited range of temperatures.

Four temperature ranges for bacteria:

1. That best at temperatures below 20°C are called psychrophiles.
2. Grows best in between 25°C and 40°C are called Mesophiles.
3. Between 45°C and 60°C thermopiles can grow.
4. Above 60 °C stenothermophiles grow best.

Bacteria

The highest population of microorganisms in a wastewater treatment plant will belong to the bacteria. They are single-called organisms which use soluble food. Conditions in the treatment plant are adjusted so that chemosererotrophs predominate. No particular species is selected as best.

Metabolism

The general tern that describes all of the chemical activities performed by a cell is metabolism. Divided into two parts.

Catabolism: Includes all the biochemical processes by which a substrate is degraded to end produces with the release of energy.

Anabolism: Includes all the biochemical processes by which the bacterium synthesizes new chemical compounds needed by the cells to hire and reproduces.

Water Microbiology

Water microbiology is concerned with the microorganisms that live in water, or can be transported from one habitat to another by water.

Water can support the growth of many types of microorganisms. This can be advantageous. For example, the chemical activities of certain strains of yeasts provide us with beer and bread. As well, the growth of some bacteria in contaminated water can help digest the poisons from the water.

However, the presence of other disease causing microbes in water is unhealthy and even life threatening. For example, bacteria that live in the intestinal tracts of humans and other warm blooded animals, such as *Escherichia coli*, *Salmonella*, *Shigella*, and *Vibrio*, can contaminate water if feces enters the water. Contamination of drinking water with a type of *Escherichia coli* known as O157:H7 can be fatal. The contamination of the municipal water supply of Walkerton, Ontario, Canada in the summer of 2000 by strain O157:H7 sickened 2,000 people and killed seven people.

The intestinal tract of warm-blooded animals also contains viruses that can contaminate water and cause disease. Examples include rotavirus, enteroviruses, and coxsackievirus.

Another group of microbes of concern in water microbiology are protozoa. The two protozoa of the most concern are *Giardia* and *Cryptosporidium*. They live normally in the intestinal tract of animals such as beaver and deer. *Giardia* and *Cryptosporidium* form dormant and hardy forms called cysts during their life cycles. The cyst forms are resistant to chlorine, which is the most popular form of drinking water disinfection, and can pass through the filters used in many water treatment plants. If ingested in drinking water they can cause debilitating and prolonged diarrhea in humans, and can be life threatening to those people with impaired immune systems. *Cryptosporidium* contamination of the drinking water of Milwaukee, Wisconsin with in 1993 sickened more than 400,000 people and killed 47 people.

Many microorganisms are found naturally in fresh and saltwater. These include bacteria, cyanobacteria, protozoa, algae, and tiny animals such as rotifers. These can be important in the food chain that forms the basis of life in the water. For example, the microbes called cyanobacteria can convert the energy of the sun into the energy it needs to live. The plentiful numbers of these organisms in turn are used as food for other life. The algae that thrive in water is also an important food source for other forms of life. A variety of microorganisms live in fresh water. The region of a water body near the shoreline (the littoral zone) is well lighted, shallow, and warmer than other regions of the water. Photosynthetic algae and bacteria that use light as energy thrive in this zone. Further away from the shore is the limnitic zone. Photosynthetic microbes also live here. As the water deepens, temperatures become colder and the oxygen concentration and light in the water decrease. Now, microbes that require oxygen do not thrive. Instead, purple and green sulphur bacteria, which can grow without oxygen, dominate. Finally, at the bottom of fresh waters (the benthic zone), few microbes survive. Bacteria that can survive in the absence of oxygen and sunlight, such as methane producing bacteria, thrive.

Saltwater presents a different environment to microorganisms. The higher salt concentration, higher pH, and lower nutrients, relative to freshwater, are lethal to many microorganisms. But, salt loving (halophilic) bacteria abound near the surface, and some bacteria that also live in freshwater are plentiful (i.e., *Pseudomonas* and *Vibrio*). Also, in 2001, researchers demonstrated that the ancient form of microbial life known as archaebacteria is one of the dominant forms of life in the ocean. The role of archaebacteria in the ocean food chain is not yet known, but must be of vital importance. Another microorganism found in saltwater are a type of algae known as dinoflagellelates. The rapid growth and multiplication of dinoflagellates can turn the water red. This "red tide" depletes the water of nutrients and oxygen, which can cause many fish to die. As well, humans can become ill by eating contaminated fish. Water can also be an ideal means of transporting microorganisms from one place to another. For example, the water that is carried in the hulls of ships to stabilize the vessels during their ocean voyages is now known to be a means of transporting microorganisms around the globe. One of these organisms, a bacterium called *Vibrio cholerae*, causes life threatening diarrhea in humans. Drinking water is usually treated to minimize the risk of microbial contamination. The importance of drinking water treatment has been known for centuries. For example, in pre-Christian times the storage of drinking water in jugs made of metal was practiced. Now, the anti-bacterial effect of some metals is known. Similarly, the boiling of drinking water, as a means of protection of water has long been known. Chemicals such as chlorine or chlorine derivatives has been a popular means of killing bacteria such as *Escherichia coli* in water since the early decades of the twentieth century. Other bacteria-killing treatments that are increasingly becoming popular include the use of a gas called ozone and the disabling of the microbe's genetic material by the use of ultraviolet light. Microbes can also be physically excluded form the water by passing the water through a filter. Modern filters have holes in them that are so tiny that even particles as miniscule as viruses can be trapped.

An important aspect of water microbiology, particularly for drinking water, is the testing of the water to ensure that it is safe to drink. Water quality testing can de done in several ways. One popular test measures the turbidity of the water. Turbidity gives an indication of the amount of suspended material in the water. Typically, if material such as soil is present in the water then microorganisms will also be present. The presence of particles even as small as bacteria and viruses can decrease the clarity of the water. Turbidity is a quick way of indicating if water quality is deteriorating, and so if action should be taken to correct the water problem. In many countries, water microbiology is also the subject of legislation. Regulations specify how often water sources are sampled, how the sampling is done, how the analysis will be performed, what microbes are detected, and the acceptable limits for the target microorganisms in the water sample. Testing for microbes that cause disease (i.e., *Salmonella typhymurium* and *Vibrio cholerae*) can be expensive and, if the bacteria are present in low numbers, they may escape detection. Instead, other more numerous bacteria provide an indication of fecal pollution of the water. *Escherichia coli* has been used as an indicator of fecal pollution for decades. The bacterium is present in the intestinal tract in huge numbers, and is more numerous than the disease-causing bacteria and viruses. The chances of detecting *Escherichia coli* is better than detecting the actual disease causing microorganisms. *Escherichia coli* also had the advantage of not being capable of growing and reproducing in the water (except in the warm and food-laden waters of tropical countries). Thus, the presence of the bacterium in water is indicative of recent fecal pollution. Finally, *Escherichia coli* can be detected easily and inexpensively.

There are two major types of water.

1. Ground water - It originates from deep wells and subterranean springs. This is virtually free of bacteria due to filtering action of soil, deep sand and rock. However, it may become contaminated when it flows along the channels.
2. Surface water - It is found in streams, lakes, and shallow wells. The air through which the rain passes may contaminate the water. Other sources are the various types of establishments and agricultural farms etc. by the sides the water flows.

Possible sources of microbial contamination of a body of water are soil and agricultural run off, farm animals, rain water, industrial waste, discharges from sewage treatment plants and storm water run off from urban areas. In water microbiology the water is contaminated when it contains a chemical or biological poison or an infectious agent. These conditions also apply to water which is polluted except that the agent or poison is often obvious and the water carries an unpleasant taste or appearance. Potability refers to the drinkability of water. When potable, it is fit for drinking. When unpotable it is unfit due to some contaminant or pollutant.

Atmospheric Waters

Rain, snow and hail which fan on land tend to carry down particles of dust, soot, and other materials suspended in the air. These often bear bacteria and other microorganisms -on their surface. The number of organisms depends upon local conditions. After heavy rain or snow the atmosphere is washed free of organisms. Surface Waters - As soon as ram or snow reaches the earth and flows over the soil, some of the soil organisms are gathered up by the water. Bodies, of water such as streams, rivers, and oceans represent surface water.

Microbial populations depend upon their numbers in the soil and, also, upon the kinds and quantities of food material dissolved out of the soil by water. Climatic, geographical and biological conditions bring about great variations in microbial populations of surface waters. Rivers and streams show their highest count during the rainy period Dust blowing into rivers and streams also contributes many microorganisms. Animals also make considerable contribution to the microbial flora of the surface waters. They bathe and often drop their excreta in the water.

Stored Waters - Inland waters held in ponds, lakes or reservoirs represent stored waters. Storage generally reduces the numbers of organisms in water. A certain degree (If purity and stability is established. Several factors affect the microbial flora of stored waters. These are as follows;

Sedimentation

Microorganisms have a specific gravity slightly greater than that of' water, and therefore slowly settle down. However, the most important factor is their attachment to suspended particles. Microorganisms are removed from the upper layers of the water as the suspended particles settle down.

Activities of other Organisms

Predatory Protozoa engulf living or dead bacteria for food, provided the water contains sufficient dissolved oxygen.

Light ray: Direct sunlight is toxic to both vegetative cells and spores of microorganisms.

The toxicity of ultraviolet rays is inversely proportional to the turbidity of water. In tropical countries direct sun light is a very effective sterilizing agent.

Temperature

Temperature has variable effects. It may kill some organisms and may stimulate the growth of others. During colder months the multiplication rate of microorganisms is considerably reduced.

Food Supply

If there is considerable vegatation or suspended food particles in the body of water, it is likely to increase the number of organisms. On the other hand, certain toxic substances may bring about marked reduction in the number of, organisms.

Ground Waters

As water seeps through the earth, microorganisms as well as suspended particles are removed by filtration in varying degrees. This depends on the permeability characteristics of the soil and the depth to which the water penetrates.

Ground water brought to the surface by springs or deep wells contains very few organisms. To construct a well the nature of the soil and underlying porous strata, the nature of the water table, and the nature, distance, and direction of the local sources of pollution must be taken into consideration.

Faecal Contamination of Water

Water gets contaminated with pathogenic microorganisms through intestinal discharges of man and animals. Further more, in the intestinal tract of man and animals, there exists a characteristic group of organism's designated as coliforms.

The coliform group of bacteria includes aerobic and facultatively anaerobic, gram negative, nonsporeforming bacilli which ferment lactose with acid and produce gas within 48 hours at, 35°C. The most common species of this group are various strains of Escherichia coli and Aerobacter aerogenes.

E. coli is commonly found in the intestinal tract of man and animals, while A. aerogenes is normally found on plants and grains, and may sometimes occur in the intestinal tract of man and animals. Contamination of water with either type makes the water unsatisfactory for drinking purposes.

Marine Microbiology

The study of microorganisms living in the sea is known as marine microbiology. Nearly three fourths of the earth's surface is covered by the sea. The sea therefore is the largest natural environment inhabited by the microorganisms. The marine environment, as does land, contains bacteria, Protozoa, algae, yeasts and moulds, as well as viruses forms organisms that live in the sea.

Microorganisms which are found in the surface layers of the sea and other aquatic environment are collectively known as plankton. Plankton may be further sub divided into phytoplank-ton (photosynthetic microorganisms, algae) and zooplankton (Protozoa, and other microscopic animals). The former are more important plankton organisms, as they arc the primary producers of organic matter. Bacteria and fungi are also present in large numbers in the plankton. Microorganisms present in the bottom regions (sediments) arc designated the benthos or benthic community. A variety of microorganisms arc found in this region. Bacteria, however, predominate.

The microbial flora characteristic of tile sea has one factor in its environmental pattern which differs from freshwater lakes, streams, and rivers, for the sea is salty. There is a high concentration of salt and mineral ions in the sea. The principal salts are the chlorides, sulphates, and carbonates of sodium, potassium, calcium and magnesium.

The concentration of dissolved salts (salinity) averages about 35 gin/kg or 3.5% by weight. Out of this 75% is NaCl. Marine microorganisms, there-fore; may be divided into two general types:

(1) those indigenous to the sea and not growing on media without sea water or high salt concentra-tion and

(2) transient organisms whose natural habitat is terrestrial and which are able to grow in media without sea water, but can tolerate high salt concentration.

There is also another group of microorganisms in the sea, in the depths of the sea microorganisms live at tremendous hydrostatic pressures, upto 1000 atmospheres. These organisms when brought to the surface require not only sea water but high pressure in order to grow. Such pressures are toxic to organisms normally living at one atmosphere at the surface.

Bacteriological Examination of Domestic Water

Natural water supplies such as rivers, lakes, and streams contain sufficient nutrients to support growth of various organisms. Microorganisms enter the water supply in several different ways. In congested centers water supplies get polluted by domestic and industrial wastes, As a potential carrier of pathogenic microorganisms, water can endanger health and life.

From the standpoint of transmitting human diseases, polluting waters with soil, rubbish, industrial wastes, and even animal manure is comparatively harmless. These sources rarely contain pathogens capable of producing human diseases when swallowed with drinking water. Sewage containing human excreta, however, is the most dangerous material that pollutes water.

People with communicable diseases of many kinds eliminate the causative organisms in their excreta. The most important microbial diseases transmitted through water are typhoid fever, paratyp-hoid fever, amoebic dysentery, bacillary dysentery, cholera, tularemia, poliomyelitis, and infectious hepatitis.

To determine the potability of water quantitative bacteriological examination may be undertaken. However, there is no single test or, even combination of tests, that is wholly satisfactory, because it will give only a fraction of the total count.

Theoretically it would be better to examine water for the presence of the specific pathogenic microorganisms. This is also impracticable because of the following reasons:

1. The methods are expensive, tedious, and slow, and by that time the water has already been consumed.
2. The number of pathogenic organisms may be quite small compared to non pathogenic organisms and would be overlooked.
3. Non-pathogenic organisms may interfere with the examination of pathogens.

The direct examination for pathogens, therefore, is not used in routine water analysis. Methods commonly used for the bacteriological examination of water, are based on:

1. The examination of presence or absence of the more common organisms of intestinal or sewage origin.
2. The approximate determination of total numbers of bacteria present in the water sample.

Microbial Components of Water

The type of microorganisms differ in unpolluted, polluted and marine waters.. In unpolluted water of mountain lake or stream there are usually low organic nutrients. The number of bacteria is very much limited, a few thousand per ml. Actinomycetes are typical. Autotrophic bacteria are common alongwith free living protozoans as Euglena, Paramecium and various amoebae.

Marine Water

The marine water is high in salt and only halophilic organisms survive. Since temperature is very low, most of them are psychrophilic. Diatoms and protozoa as dinoflagellates are important components in food chain. In the off shore oceanic zone, photosynthetic organisms are present. These are diatoms and dinoflagellates.

Most marine microbes are found along the shoreline or littoral zone where nutrients are in abundance. Some unusual types are also present on the ocean floor in the benthic zone and even at the bottom of several miles-deep trenches, the abyssal zone.

Polluted Water

In polluted waters, there are large amounts of organic matter from sewage, feces and industrial complex. The microbes are usually heterotrophic. The digestion of organic matter by these organisms is incomplete, due to which there accumulate acids, bases, alcohols and various gases.

The major type of bacteria are coliform bacteria the Gram-negative nonsporeforming bacilli usually found in the intestine. This group includes E. coli and species of Enterabacter. They ferment lactose to acid and gas. Noncoliform bacteria Streptococcus, Proteus and Pseudomonas are also present. Under some conditions, the polluting organisms multiply rapidly and consume most of the available oxygen. For instance, nutrients enter the river from sources like sewage treatment plants or urban suburban runoff.

Thus river suddenly develops a high nutrient content. Under these conditions algae may bloom rapidly. This leads to depletion of oxygen in water. There is very little oxygen available to the protozoa, small animals, fish and plants. Due to this non-availability of oxygen, a layer of dead organisms, mud and silt accumulate at the bottom, and anaerobeic species of Clostridium, Desulfovibrio etc. will flourish. They produce gases. One gas, H2S combines with lead or iron to give a precipitate which makes the mud black and the water poisonous. Due to complete depletion of oxygen, the suspended bacteria die in their own waste products. There is hardly any life in water at this stage. The gas bubbles from the anaerobes in the mud break the surface. Such processes lead to death of a river.

Water Pollution

Polluted waters can be classified in different ways. In microbiological context, there are generally recognised physical, chemical and biological pollution of water.

Physical Water Pollution

Here the water becomes cloudy due to presence of some particulate matter such as sand or soil. Some plant material as algal-bloom may also be involved, that turns the consistency of water like a pea soup. Presence of some phosphates or nitrates may encourage the growth of blooms leading finally to a condition known as eutrophication. This upsets the ecological balance.

Chemical Water Pollution

It occurs due to introduction of inorganic and organic waste to water. For example, water passing out of a mine contains large amount of copper, iron or other ore. Another source of pollution is metal pipelines. Corrosion of metals of the pipes may yield rusty or black precipitates. Other chemical pollutants include laundry detergents, radioactive wastes and nitrates from fertilisers etc. An important group of chemicals are polychlorinated biphenyls or PCBs, a group of industrial chemicals used in the production of electric insulators and paper products. They are carcinogenic and necessary to be eliminated from water. Main sources of chemical pollutants are mining wastes, air pollutants (washed down by rain), power plants, industries, sewage and storm water runoff, wash from farm lands (pesticides, fertilisers), hospitals, road salts and exhausts from automobiles.

Biological Water Pollution

It develops from the microorganisms that enter waters from such sources as human waste, food operations, meat packing plants and medical facilities etc. Under normal conditions, the water body is able to handle biological material, because heterotrophs digest the organic matter to simple phosphates, nitrates and sulphates which fertilise the plants. Carbohydrates are converted to CO2 and water, which are also useful to plants. The plants then release °2 through photosynthesis. Due to rapid movement of water, aeration is more or less constant and the wastes eliminated.

However, there arises the problem when water becomes stagnant or is overloaded with waste. Water is now unable to handle the biological material, and it soon becomes polluted. We have already seen how a lake may turn into a swamp due to overabundance of organic matter. A critical factor operating under such a situation is the biological oxygen demand (BOD). It refers to the oxygen requirement by the metabolising organisms. As the number of organisms increases, the demand for 02 increases proportionally. Depletion of 02 in water may lead to death of fish and other aquatic animals, a flat taste of water, and eventual death of aerobes.

The BOD is therefore an important indication of the levels of biological pollution in the water. In laboratory, BOD is determined by measuring the amount of dissolved oxygen in test samples of water distributed to BOD bottles. Initial determination of dissolved oxygen in sample is made. The bottles are then stoppered and incubated at 20°C for five days, after which the amount of dissolved oxygen is again determined. The difference in the oxygen content represents the amount of oxygen used up in the test sample, which is the BOD. Results are expressed as parts per million (ppm). A BOD of several hundred is taken usually high.

Diseases Transmitted by Water

Water is infact a vehicle for the transfer of a wide range of diseases of microbial origin. The important bacterial diseases include typhoid fever, cholera and bacterial dysentry that are generally transmitted when human feces from carriers or patients contaminates the water. Viral diseases transmitted by water include virus A hepatitis and polio. Many protozoa form cysts which survive for long periods in water. The causal agents of amoebiasis, giardiasis etc. are important concerns in water pollution.

Water Treatment

We have seen that water and sewage harbour a variety of organisms responsible for diseases in man. It is thus necessary to remove or rather interrupt the disease cycle in nature through treatment of water and sewage. Water purification and sanitary sewage disposal are two major methods for interrupting disease cycle. In water purification organisms are prevented from reaching the body whereas in sewage disposal, they are removed from body waste products. The various steps in the purification of drinking water in municipal water supplies are, It may be seen that there are three basic steps in the purification of drinking water: sedimentation, filtration and chlorination.

Sedimentation Process

Water usually undergoes some degree of purification during storage in ponds or reservoirs. Suspended particles settle and carry down most of the microorganisms. The rate of purification by sedimentation depends upon the kind and amount of suspended matter as the well as physical, chemical and biological conditions of the stored water. The rate of sedimentation is enhanced by adding alum, iron salts, colloidal silicate, etc., which produce flocculent precipitates. Microorganisms and suspended particles are entrapped and settle rapidly. Sometimes activated carbon is also added. This adsorbs the compound responsible for objectionable colour and taste of water. Microorganisms remain viable for a considerable time, even though visible evidence of pollution has disappeared. Sedimentation, therefore, reduces the microbial population but does not sterilize polluted water. To produce potable water further treatment is necessary. Thus sedimentation is often used as a first stage purification.

Filtration Process

This process removes the remaining microorganisms from the water. Although, different types of filter material are available, mostly a layer of sand and gravel is utilised to trap the microorganisms. A slow sand filter uses several feet deep layer of fine sand particles. Within the sand there forms a layer of microorganisms which acts as an additional filter. This layer is called a Schmutzdecke or dirty layer. To cleanse the filter, the top layer is removed and replaced with fresh sand. A rapid sand filter contains coarser particles of gravel. The schmutzdecke does not develop; the filtration rate is higher (over 200 million gallons per acre per day). This type of filter is generally used in municipal supplies.

Slow Sand Filter

Slow sand filtration plants require considerable area because the rate of filtration is slow. A concrete floor with drainage tiles to collect the filtered water is constructed. The tile is covered with coarse gravel, fine gravel, coarse sand and finally 2 to 1 feet of sand at the top. Water seeps through the filter slowly., is collected by tile drain pipes at the bottom, and is pumped into a reservoir. At best five million gallons of water per acre, per day, can be filtered. Slow sand filters are clogged by turbid water. Water to be filtered is, therefore, clarified by sedimentation with or without coagulation.

The purification of water is accomplished not by the screening action of the sand for the spaces arc much to large, but by a different principle. A colloidal, flocculent material composed of bacteria, algae, and Protozoa accumulates in the surface layers of fine sand. This Slimy, gelatinous film closes up the pores between the sand grains and makes the filter bed more and more effective. Since bacteria have a negative electrical charge and colloidal material on the sand grains has a. positive charge, bacteria are thus adsorbed on the particles.

Bacteria arc also injested by Protozoa that Inhabit the upper layer of the film. Metabolic activity of microorganisms also greatly reduces the chemical content of the water. When, the gelatinous film finally become too thick, the efficiency of the filter gradually decreases. The filter is taken out of service and the surface layer is cleaned.

Rapid Sand Filter

Rapid sand filters are constructed in a manner similar to that of slow sand filters. They also consist of layers of sand, gravel, and rock. Water is pretreated before filtration by a coagulant such as alum or ferrous sulphate. The water passes through a settling tank in which most of thc precipitate settles out, and the remainder is pumped on to the filter. Rapid sand filters soon become clogged and are cleaned by forcing cleaned water backward (back washed) through the bed of gravel and sand, and bubbling air through them.

The back water rises through the filter and carries the accumulated material to the sewer. The wash water is thus wasted, Care is taken in this backwashing procedure to see that the fine sand on the surface is not lost. Rapid sand filters are usually operated in batteries, so that some may be in operation, while others are being cleaned.

They are nearly as effective as slow sand filters but operate 50 times faster than slow sand filters. Rapid sand filters are capable of delivering 150 to 200 million gallons of water per acre, per day. They require a much smaller area of land for more water filtrations and cost much less to install and maintain.

Many other filtration devices such as pressure filters, diatomite fitters, membrane filter, reverse osmosis etc, are employed to remove various impurities in water. Recovery of potable water from the sea and from domestic and. industrial sewage is also undertaken by the use of filtration techniques.

Chlorination Process

In this final step, chlorine gas is added to the water. This gas is an active oxidant which reacts with organic matter in the water. Gas is added until any residue is present. A residue of 0.2 ppm-1.0 ppm of water is often the standard used. Under these conditions, most remaining microbes die within 30 minutes.

Bacteriological Analysis of Water

There are methods to detect bacterial contamination of water. The chief objective is to identify coliform organisms as Escherichia coli. Their presence indicates that water contains fecal pollution and is unsafe for consumption.

Membrane Filter Technique

It may be used in the field also. A special, collecting bottle is held against the water current and a 100-ml sample is taken. The water is filtered through a membrane filter and the filter pad is then transferred to a plate of bacteriological medium. Bacteria trapped in the filter will form colonies which may be counted.

Standard Plate Count SPC

Water sample is diluted in sterile buffer. Measured amounts are pipetted into Petri dishes. Agar medium is added and plates incubated. Colony counts are made and multiplied by the reciprocal dilution factor to have total bacteria per ml water. This method is similar to that used for milk.

Most Propable Number

In this procedure, water in 10 ml, I mi and 0.1 mt amounts is inoculated into lactose broth tubes. The tubes are incubated and coliform organisms may be identified by their production of gas from the lactose. By referring to a MPN table, a statistical range of the number of coliform may be determined by observing how many broth tubes showed gas. This method does not detect total number of bacteria in the water nor it locate noncoliforms like Salmonella. However it indicates the presence and quantity of coliforms.

Specific Tests For Asseing Water Coliform Counts

The most frequently used indicator organism is the normally nonpathogenic Coliform bacterium Escherichia coli. Positive tests for E. coli do not prove the presence of enteropathogens, such as Salmonella and Shigella, but do establish the possibility. E. coli is more numerous and easier to be grown.

Presumptive Test

A series of lactose broth or lauryl sulphate tryptose broth fermentation tubes are inoculated with measured amounts of water and incubated at 35°C for 24 to 48 hours. The formation of gas in the inverted vial in the fermentation tube within 48 hours indicates a positive presumptive test. Absence of gas formation at the end of 48 hours constitutes a negative presumptive test. This means that the water sample does not contain coliforms and is considered safe.

Confirmed Test

Sometimes a false positive presumptive test is obtained. This may be due to the presence of yeasts, certain Clostridium species and some other organisms, or by bacterial associations or synergism. In order to be certain that gas-production is due to coliforms a confirmed test must be performed.

Two procedures are normally employed. In one method a drop of culture from a positive lactose broth tube is transferred to brilliant green lactose bile fermentation broth, and is incubated for 24 to 48 hours at 35°C. The appearance of gas within 48 hrs constitues a positive confirmed test.

The dye inhibits gram positive organisms and eliminates a false presumptive test and the syngergistic reaction of gram positive and gram negative organisms growing together. In the second method a drop of culture from the positive lactose broth is streaked on a petriplate containing, Endo's, or eosin-methylene blue agar. The appearance of nucleated colonies, with or without a metallic sheen, within 24 hours indicates a positive confirmed test.

Completed Test

Isolated colonies from petriplates are transferred into lactose fermentation broth and streaked on to an agar slant. The presence of gas in the fermentation broth and the presence of gram negative non spore-forming bacilli on the slant give evidence that coliform bacteria were present in the original water sample.

IMViC Reaction

E. coli and A. aerogenes are normally referred to as faecal and non-faecal contaminants of water, respectively, and are the most important organisms of the coliform group. Since they closely resemble each other in their morphological and cultural characteristics, biochemical tests, are, performed to differentiate them. These tests are collectively designated as the IMViC reactions. The name was coined by Parr from the first letters of the four tests, namely Indole, Methyl red, Voges Proskauer, and Citrate. There are 16 possible combinations of positive and negative tests of these four characteristics. Most, of these combinations have been found, but the reactions of E. coli and A. aerogenes are commonly found. The remaining 14 types are usually designated as "intermediates".

Aquatic Microbes: Impact on Man and Environment

The aquatic environment is that part of the earth covered with water and it is alled the hydrosphere. Air is the atmosphere while soil is the lithosphere. ydrosphere, atmosphere and lithosphere comprise the biosphere, i.e. an nvironment where living things are found. Microbes are minute living hings that occur in all environments and are therefore ubiquitous. The environment has received more attention globally and locally in the last decade after the United Nations Earth Summit in Rio de Janeiro, 1992. As Professor of Environmental Microbiology, the biosphere is my research domain. But of particular interest to me is the hydrosphere, my specialty being aquatic microbial ecology and water pollution. So, I have chosen for my inaugural lecture the topic, "Aquatic microbes: impact on man and environment".

Microorganisms in the aquatic environment affect man either positively or negatively, directly or indirectly. In other words, these minute living things may be beneficial or harmful to man, his activities as well as other natural resources. For purposes of completeness, it is noted that the presence of some microorganisms in water may sometimes have no apparent or visible effect, being neutral to the ecosystem.

The ecosystem is the highest organization in the hierarchy of life. It covers individual organisms in the food chain, populations, energy flow, biogeochemical cycles, interactions between living and non- living resources, as well as human impact. Microorganisms are involved in all of these activities hence man should take cognizance of microorganisms in sustainable development.

Discovery of Microorganisms

For a long time man was not aware of the existence of the microbial world. At that time, activities and impacts of microbes were attributed to the supernatural. The reason is not far fetched. A microbe is invisible to the unaided human eye. In other words our limit of vision does not cover the size of a microbe. We can all visualize one metre length, one centimetre i.e. one hundredth of a metre. But a smaller division of a metre such as one millionth or billionth is not discernable by the unaided human eye. Thanks to Physics and the advent of magnifying lenses. The microscope is used to enlarge cells so that the morphology or shape of a microbial cell can be discerned. It was Antony van Leewenhoeck (1677) who in 1676 made crude microscopes and, out of curiosity, used them to examine various specimens including well- and sea- water. He discovered what he called 'animacules' or 'minute animals'. van Leewenhoeck thus initiated the study of aquatic microbes and is indeed the father of Environmental Microbiology. Whereas a bacterial cell is not visible by the naked human eye, a population of bacteria may become visible after the individual cells are cultured having been supplied with nutrients for growth and multiplication to the size of a mass of cells or a colony. Even today, it is not easy to appreciate and acknowledge the presence of microorganisms. Man tends to relate to the effect, result or symptoms produced by the activities of microorganisms.

What of fermentation of palm juice into palm wine (Odeyemi & Akpata,1988)? Salmonellosis contracted from poultry (Akpata & Fashola, 1985)? Anyone would give prompt attention to gastroenteritis (upset stomach) from cholera or dysentery due to drinking contaminated water or eating molluscs harvested from a polluted bay. If microorganisms cause changes that are pleasant, the process is maintained, if undesirable or harmful, the process is terminated or controlled.

Position of Aquatic Microbes in the Evolution of Life

Let us look at microbes in water, their evolution and niches. Water as a chemical (H2O) is devoid of carbon/energy and nitrogen sources of nutrients required for the growth of living things. It is the presence of extraneous substances in water that provides the nutrients for microbial growth. These microbes affect the quality of water and thereby influence the use that man makes of it.

There are microorganisms in water. Some are indigenous to water and are called autochthonous species while some are foreign or allochthonous species that find their way into the aquatic environment. Autochthonous species are involved in the cleansing of water, utilizing the little nutrients available because a clean body of water is referred to as oligotrophic, having low nutrient content. When wastes are loaded into water it becomes eutrophic providing nutrients for microbial proliferation. In this way, eutrophication causes ecosystem dis-equilibrium, initiating signs of pollution with ultimate loss of the value of the aquatic resources. Water is an essential natural resource for sustainability of life. It is known that a living organism requires water at some stage of its life cycle: the human, the developing embryo or foetus, the mosquito larva, the germinating plant seed or microbial spore requires water for survival. Some arid lands require only irrigation for vegetation to develop!

Indeed the abundant water on the surface of planet Earth millions of years ago, was the conducive environment for the formation of molecules into the cytoplasmic broth that constituted the precursors of the first living things.These led to the evolution of the primitive cell (protocaryote) or prokaryote in which the nucleus is naked. Is it not interesting that bacteria and bluegreen algae belong to this group? The eucaryotic cell of fungi, protozoa and indeed multicellular organisms, including man, evolved later with a nuclear membrane and more complex organisation. It is noteworthy that the biochemical activities of microorganisms contributed a lot to the maintenance of an oxygen atmosphere responsible for the existence of life on earth.

Thus, microorganisms evolved in water and to date various species remain in their habitat of origin occupying different niches in the aquatic environment. Microbes abound in surface waters: fresh, brackish and marine. They occur in rivers, lakes, estuaries and the seas. By their microscopic size and versatile metabolic capabilities, microbes find niches and can colonize the biosphere. The number of microorganisms in surface waters is high because of the input from natural, and anthropogenic (manmade) sources including various industries. During rainfall, natural run-off washes soil microorganisms into rivers and streams that become turbid.

Also, urbanization creates large populations that generate wastes e.g. refuse (solid) and sewage (liquid). The disposal of these waste materials remains a colossal problem. There is the urbanization of farm animals and general agricultural practices including irrigation of crops that also contribute to increased number of microorganisms in water.

Bacteria are found in the shores and depths of the seas including the hypersaline dead sea with salinity above 35%o (parts per thousand). These are the extremely halophilic bacteria e.g. *Halobacterium halobium* (Haruhico *et al.*(1995). Research on halophiles has contributed to understanding the activities of osmophilic bacteria in the preservation of food with salt or sugar. Microbes get adapted to environmental changes or challenges by the modification of their metabolic pathways and evolution of genetic apparatus required to meet the demands of the new situation. This knowledge is exploited by man in the production of microbial metabolites like antibiotics, and in genetic engineering of microbes for specific characters.

The isolation of microbes from aquatic thermal vents opened a new vista for producing industrial enzymes that are stable at high temperatures (100?C). Therefore, denaturation of enzymes is avoided and the cost of cooling to protect mesophilic enzymes is saved. Eveleigh and others at Cook College of Rutgers University, USA elucidated the enzyme of an extremophilic bacterium. I had the privilege of working with Douglas Eveleigh during my last sabbatical leave.

Water also occurs underground in water tables or aquifers having percolated through the soil layers. Hence, spring water arising from the aquifer is ordinarily clear and palatable. However, seepage of effluents in refuse dumps and other human activities involving the subsurface of the earth aggravate the contamination of ground water thus interfering with the quality of spring water. Microorganisms in ground water constitute a health hazard to consumers. In a setting with little or irregular supply of pipe-borne water and usually, well water quality is not tested, consumers are vulnerable to waterborne infections. It is the scarcity of potable water that has enhanced the sale of the so-called 'pure 'water sachets. For safety of packaged drinking water in Nigeria, the activities of the National Agency for Food Drug Administration Control (NAFDAC) deserve commendation. As an environmentalist, I would add that the used sachets constitute a nuisance especially as the waste is recalcitrant, and being non-biodegradable, it is persistent in the environment. Furthermore, care needs to be taken about the location of disposal sites for solid wastes.

The geology of the underlying soil should be considered and the disposal site may be lined before dumping, and the refuse covered with an impervious material. These efforts would control wetting of refuse by rainfall and mitigate the seepage of effluents into the aquifer with its eventual contamination and negative impact on consumers.

Water Pollution

The aquatic environment has a natural ability for self-purification. Physicochemical and biologic activities including microbiologic action bring about the breakdown of small quantities of organic materials. In effect, contaminated body of water such as a stream can be cleansed through selfpurification processes (Akpata, 1998).

It is when the type of waste is nonbiodegradable e.g. plastics or the amount of organic input exceeds the carrying capacity of the environment that there emanate undesirable conditions that elicit negative impacts on the ecosystem. This is the stage that there is environmental pollution.

Faecal Pollution of Lagos Lagoon

A trip using the famous UNILAG 1, motorboat of the erstwhile Department of Biological Sciences, was undertaken to survey the Lagos lagoon for areas of point source pollution. Nobody could ignore Iddo site of faeces disposal for the stench and unaesthetic value. There was a need to enquire from the Lagos City Council just what was going on? Iddo is located on the Lagos Mainland and is accessible to Mushin, Yaba, Ebute- Metta, Surulere, and so on. The faeces point was near the Carter Bridge on the mainland end. The rationale for disposal of raw faeces into the Lagos lagoon at Iddo was that the waste would be washed into the sea and diluted to extinction. In that case, the waste would not be seen and there would be no visible or apparent impact on the aquatic ecosystem.

To clarify the situation, a research study was designed to investigate the distribution of faeces in the lagoon. Samples of fresh faeces obtained from the disposal vehicle or lagoon water were cultured for pathogens and commensals. The Lagos City Council recorded the volumes of faeces deposited into the lagoon. Seven sampling stations were identified on the lagoon, some were located to the north while others were to the south of the faeces disposal point. An apparently unpolluted station located in the middle of the lagoon served as control. Some physicochemical parameters e.g. temperature, pH, salinity, suspended organic matter and turbidity were measured at each sampling station. Faecal pollution was assayed using faecal indicator bacteria namely, coliforms, *Escherichia coli, Streptococcus faecalis or Clostridium perfringes* for their value in determining the period of pollution. Vertical and horizontal distribution of faecal bacteria in the lagoon was studied at each sampling station so as to determine the abundance and distribution of faeces in the aquatic ecosystem.

The results showed presence of pathogens e.g. *Salmonella* and *Shigella* species in the faeces samples from some areas. However, pathogens were not isolated from stations on the lagoon. It was observed that *Escherichia coli* count decreased rapidly southwards near the sea and less rapidly northwards nearer Ogun River (Akpata & Ekundayo, 1978). It is probable that stations where faecal bacteria were isolated had been contaminated with faeces and possibly pathogens. There was both horizontal and vertical distribution of faeces in the lagoon. Higher counts of bacteria were obtained in bottom samples an indication that sedimentation of faeces occurred at each station. This could be due to the effect of gravity and increased organic nutrients. Twenty-six million litres of faeces were deposited into the lagoon at Iddo in 1973. Our results showed that the faeces were not always washed southwards into the sea from the Lagos lagoon as suggested by the Lagos City Council.

Movement of Faeces in the Lagoon

Other factors, e.g. meteorological that could affect the distribution of faeces in the lagoon were considered. Records were obtained of the tide levels and our times of collecting samples. The faeces were washed southwards into the sea at low tide. During high tide however, faeces were washed northwards i.e. hinterland towards Ogun River. It is sad to note that Ogun River is one of the sources of raw water for purification at the water works. Increased contamination of the raw water puts pressure on the facilities for the purification of potable water distributed through a network of pipes to Lagos metropolis for domestic and other uses. So, movement of water in the lagoon affects other bodies of water that are connected. Our results elucidated the significance of pollution of Lagos lagoon with faeces and the negative impact of this process on the maintenance of a balanced ecological milieu of the lagoon and similar aquatic environments. Therefore, the choice of Iddo as location for dumping faeces lacked a sound scientific scrutiny.

Investigations on Sawdust Pollution of Lagos Lagoon

At Ebute Metta, Okobaba, there are sawmills located on the bank of the lagoon. Logs of timber are floated on the lagoon at this station. Sawdust generated from milling the logs is heaped beside the lagoon. The heaps were washed by water during wave action and current into the lagoon. At this station, the occurrence and periodicity of fungi in Lagos lagoon were studied with a view to understanding the ecology of fungi and their roles in the biodegradation of the plant material polluting the lagoon. In contrast, the biological pollutant at Iddo station was of animal origin and our investigations were mainly on the bacteriological status of the lagoon.

Bacteria and fungi are major groups of microorganisms in the aquatic ecosystem. Samples of water were collected aseptically from designated stations on the lagoon and analyzed for fungi using different culture media. Some physicochemical features e.g. depth, turbidity, temperature, pH, total suspended solids, dissolved oxygen and salinity of the lagoon were measured during sample collection to see if there were correlations with the occurrence of fungi. Some fungi occurred throughout the year whereas others appeared seasonally (Akpata & Ekundayo, 1983). Members of the genus *Mucor* occurred during the rainy season or at stations having low salinity as recorded at mid-lagoon. The Lagos lagoon was shallow at the sawdust station; values for turbidity and suspended solids were high whereas dissolved oxygen level was low. Salinity varied with season, being higher in the dry season, lower during the rains and at the mid-lagoon control station.

The implications of these results were explained by carrying out some laboratory studies.

Environmental Impact Assessment (EIA)

Environmental Impact Assessment (EIA) is an evaluation usually carried out by a multidisciplinary team of experts and the results are of predictive value. Thus, it is best to perform an EIA prior to the establishment of a project. The team writes an Environmental Impact Statement (EIS) on the proposed project so that an appropriate decision can be made by policy makers on the suitability of the project at that location. If projects have been implemented however, an EIA would reveal their impacts on the environment and suggest measures to mitigate negative consequences.

Most of our research work conducted in this area in the 1970s contributed to an ecological auditing of the aquatic habitats. Data obtained on the microbiota of Lagos lagoon constituted a baseline for future investigations as there was no available literature of such studies previously. Briefly our work at the Iddo faeces disposal site showed that movement of the waste matter was determined by several factors. Sometimes faeces were not washed into the sea and diluted to extinction as proposed. The organic load was beyond the self-purification ability of the lagoon ecosystem. So, there was habitat change with a shift in population from normal aerobic biota of clean water to allochthonous populations including Enterobacteriaceae and anaerobic microorganisms. Anaerobic metabolism produces incomplete decomposition of substrates with volatile metabolites that may have bad smell (Ekundayo, 1977). Continual loading of the lagoon overwhelmed the aquatic ecosystem resulting in an ecological imbalance with consequent signs of pollution. Thus rehabilitation of the lagoon was indicated.

EIA on the Lagos Lagoon

In a collaborative study with Oyenekan & Nwankwo, the impacts of biological pollutants in the Lagos lagoon on the algae, bacteria and benthic invertebrates were investigated (Akpata *et al.*1993). Sawdust caused silting and oxygen deficient water. Organic matter content of the lagoon had a direct correlation with the coliform and heterotrophic bacterial populations but was negatively correlated with benthic fauna. Biological pollutants in Lagos lagoon imposed turbidity that reduced depth of light penetration with consequent decrease in photosynthetic activities including dissolved oxygen concentration. Therefore, pollution has negative impacts on primary and secondary production of the aquatic ecosystem.

Sewage Treatment at Agbara Industrial Estate

Agbara Industrial Estate is sited in Ogun State near Lagos. There are many industries providing different products and services. Also, many residential buildings were located within the estate. Our interest was on the management of waste waters in the estate. The activities in the estate generate both domestic sewage and industrial waste waters carried in sewers (pipes) to a central sewage treatment plant. Here, there was controlled mixing of waste waters in tanks in which the activated sludge method of sewage treatment was employed. In a collaborative study with Nwachukwu and Essien, it was demonstrated that mixing of domestic and industrial sewage enhanced biodegradation of the waste and the treated effluent had lower microbial load than raw sewage (Nwachukwu *et al.,*1990).

Our work on Agbara sewage treatment facility confirmed that treatment of sewage produced effluent with less organic load that can be degraded by the autochthonous microorganisms as part of the self-purification process of the receiving environment. In contrast, at Iddo, there was no prior treatment of raw human faeces, poured into the Lagos lagoon, so there was excess organic load or nutrient consequently, deterioration of the quality of water ensued and all signs of water pollution were evident.

Studies on Owo River

The work on Owo River was by a team of experts in various disciplines, namely; hydrology, algalogy, benthic ecology, chemistry, sanitary engineering and microbiology.

Our studies on the hydrobiology of Owo River revealed the algae and microorganisms (Nwankwo *et al.*, 1999). The populations of the organisms were recorded thus providing qualitative and quantitative data on the ecological auditing of the aquatic environment. The effort of the Lagos state government in laying baseline data on an important water source is acknowledged. These data will serve as references for EIA of projects that might impact on Owo River in future.

Reports from other Countries

The presence of microorganisms as a result of pollution with biological waste could have negative impacts on man as well as on the ecology of the body of water leading to morbidity and mortality of aquatic living resources. For example, the massive fish kill in the Gulf coincided with the proliferation of a bacterium, *Streptococcus iniae* (EPA Report, 2001). Also, Evison (1985) reported that sewage in water could contaminate shellfish and bathers in affected beaches may run the risk of infection.

Sewage Disposal in Newcastle-upon-Tyne, UK

This was the work done in 1983 during my visit to the Public Health Section, Department of Civil Engineering, University of Newcastle- upon-Tyne, England. In collaboration with Lilian Evison we investigated the relationship of protozoa to bacterial populations in different sites where sewage passed from the treatment plant at Howden to the River Tyne. Cultural and microscopic methods were used to assess bacterial populations. Direct epifluorescent microsopic examination was employed in studying the protozoa in the laboratory (Hobbie *et al.,* 1977). The domestic sewage from Newcastle- upon - Tyne metropolis was treated at Howden. There was an inverse relationship between bacterial counts and protozoa populations. The treated effluent had reduced microbial counts an indication of lower organic matter content. The sludge, in which most of the polluting materials were concentrated, was loaded into a boat that carried the waste far into the sea for disposal.

Experiences gained in Newcastle-upon-Tyne and Agbara Industrial Estate emphasize the advantages of sewage treatment in maintaining balanced ecological status of an aquatic environment. Indeed the treatment facility should be monitored to ensure that it performs efficiently so that both effluent and sludge will have no detrimental effect on the environment.

Impact of Water Hyacinth on Nigerian Coastal Waters

In discussing the importance of EIA, I would like us to mention water hyacinth, and to highlight the contribution, in 1985, of the University of Lagos team of experts to the 'Invasion of Lagos waters by water hyacinth, *Eichhornia crassipes* Mart.' (Kusemiju *et al.*1987). Members of the team were: Kusemiju, Okusanya, Akpata and Oyenekan. The source of the weed was traced by boat from Lagos to the border with the Republic of Benin. The EIA was well documented and predictions have come to realization.

Namely, that the plant was a strange weed in Lagos waters; that it loves fresh waters; and that its rate of proliferation would hasten its colonization of our rivers and streams. Short term, medium term and long-term measures to control the spread of the weed were recommended. Policy decision was slow and implementation of recommendations was not forthcoming. Here is a good example of the gap between research findings, government policy and implementation. Now, the weed is a problem in many aquatic systems in Nigeria (Kusemiju *et al.*1988).

Complimentality of Laboratory Experimentation to Field Observations

There were differences observed between sea, lagoon and river water in their physicochemical properties and microbial contents. So, various experiments were set up in the laboratory to elucidate our findings in these aquatic environments. Further experiments were performed on the roles of microbes in nutrient cycling in the aquatic ecosystem.

Effects of Seawater on Indicator Bacteria

Laboratory experiments were set up to study survival of bacteria in the lagoon (Akpata *et al., 1979;* Amund *et al., 1982).* Bacteria of enteric origin are allochthonous to the Lagos lagoon. However these are the standard faecal indicators. We were not unmindful of the effect on these bacteria, of the prevailing physicochemical factors in the lagoon. This explained the importance of the studies on the ecology of the microorganisms in the aquatic ecosystem.

The Lagos lagoon is an estuary that opens into the Atlantic Ocean. Some rivers flow into the lagoon. The sea has high salt content being made up of different ionic components e.g. Na+, Ca++, Mg++, Cl-, CO3—, SO4—. On the contrary, river water has few ions, low salinity hence it is fresh to drink. Differences in the physicochemical factors of rivers and the lagoon would affect the microbial populations that can impact on the self-purification ability of the aquatic environments.

Salinity of the lagoon varied seasonally and from station to station. The effect of salinity and ionic concentrations on the distribution of the bacteria was studied with a view to contributing to our understanding of the distribution and survival of faecal bacteria in the lagoon (Akpata *et al.*1979).

Salinity had a negative impact on the cells of *Escherichia coli.* Microscopic studies revealed large numbers of the cells in varying sizes. Laboratory experiments showed that faecal bacteria had improved survival pattern in presence of organic nutrients. It was suggested that the higher organic matter content recorded at the northern stations and at bottom samples favoured the survival of indicator bacteria. It was also noted that the sedimentation of biological pollutants enriched the bottom of the lagoon and this enhanced survival of bacteria by their protection from damage or injury.

Effect of Sunlight and Ultra Violet Irradiation on Faecal Bacteria

Being a tropical country with abundant sunlight hours and intensity, we sought to investigate the impact of sunlight or ultraviolet radiation on the bacteria in the lagoon. In a collaborative study with Ekundayo and Oguntuyo (now Dr (Mrs) Aboaba), a laboratory experiment was set up using light and dark regimes on enteric pathogens namely; *Escherichia coli, Salmonella typhi* and *Shigella flexneri* (Ekundayo *et al.*, 1978). The research revealed that exposure of some enteric bacteria to sunlight or ultra violet irradiation had a negative impact on their survival and elucidated the survival pattern of some bacteria in tropical water. It is known that UV light causes dimerisation of DNA molecules thus impairing growth (Davies & Evison, 1991). From this work it was evident that paucity of bacteria at the seaward station was influenced by both the chemical composition of seawater and the damaging effect of sunlight on the cells.

Salinity and light are stress- inducing factors for enteric bacteria in the Lagos lagoon. Our observation was later explained by the phenomenon of viable but nonculturable bacteria (Colwell *et al.*,1985). Under unfavourable environmental conditions, spore - forming bacteria produce endospores and could remain dormant for a long time! The faecal indicator bacteria employed in this study were of the coliform group being Gram negative, non-spore forming rods. Their vegetative cells are affected by the prevailing conditions and the stress- induced bacteria become debilitated. Thus the cells cannot perform physiological functions but they remain viable i.e. alive being in a state of ill health. At this point an attempt to culture or grow the cells on ordinary laboratory media fails. It would then appear that the bacteria were not present in the sample. Nonculturable bacteria may be included in assays using Acridine Orange Direct Count (AODC) reported by Hobbie *et al.* (1977). The bacteria would require to be resuscitated before growth can occur in laboratory media.

Salinity Tolerance of Fungi Isolated from Lagos Lagoon

The effect of salt content on fungal growth and sporulation in the lagoon was investigated. The results indicated that fungi e.g. *Cladosporium sp.* that occurred throughout the year tolerated a wide range of salinities. Members of the *Mucorales* that occurred only in the rainy season grew and sporulated only at low salinities below 5 ‰ (Akpata & Ekundayo,1983).

Effects of Sawdust on Germination of Fungal Spores in Lagos Lagoon

The effects of wood extracts on fungal spore germination and germ tube lengths were measured. Information was obtained on the types of wood species transported on the lagoon. Aqueous extracts were prepared of sawdust of wood species namely; *Khaya ivorensis (iroko), Mitragyna ciliata (abura) and Triplochiton scleroxylon(obeche).* Laboratory experiments were designed such that spores of different fungi were incubated in wood extracts. Aliquots of the cultures were examined with the microscope and quantitative data were obtained on number of spores germinated. Also, lengths of germ tubes were measured with a calibrated eyepiece micrometer inserted in a microscope (Akpata, 1987). Length of germ tube and number of spores germinated increased significantly for *Aspergillus flavus* in the extract of *K. ivorensis*. This contributed to the population of the fungus in the aquatic ecosystem.

Microscopic Examination of the Architecture of Conidiophores of Aspergillus Iganteus

One of the fungi isolated from the sawdust pollution site was *Aspergillus giganteus* that has very tall and slim conidiophores. The internal structure of the conidiophores was examined microscopically using birefringence and dichroism. The knowledge could be useful to or impact positively on the architecture and engineering design of slim and tall buildings. Part of this work was carried out in the laboratory of Graham Gooday at the Department of Biochemistry and Molecular Biology, Marischal College, Aberdeen, UK.

Studies on Bioconversion and Degradation of Waste Materials in Coastal Evironments

The ability of fungi to degrade cellulose, a major component of wood was tested in laboratory experiments. The findings elucidated the roles of fungi in the lagoon ecosystem. For example, some fungi participated in the decomposition of wood wastes in Lagos lagoon. An unidentified basidiomycotina grew and produced fruiting body on sawdust. Also, *Aspergillus species and Trichoderma aureoviride* breakdown filter paper cellulose in laboratory experiments. Fungi thus participate in the biogeochemical cycling of substances in the environment. Cellulose degrading fungi produced enzyme cellulases that may be useful in various industries.

Another biodegradation study was carried out using chitin, component of the shell of shrimp, squid and other animals, an abundant waste in the aquatic environment. Unlike cellulose which is a aliphatic polymer of glucose units, chitin is an aromatic polymer of N-acetylglucosamine units and the presence of a benzene ring makes the molecule more stable and difficult to attack by microorganisms. Bioconversion of chitin by some estuarine bacteria was investigated with a view to finding a natural production of chitosan that is of demand in pharmaceutical and other industries (Akpata,1993). Harsh chemical methods are used in the production of commercial chitosan

Molecular Biology Approach to Environmental Microbiology

Just as the advent of magnifying lenses opened a new area in scientific knowledge and research into the hitherto unknown world of microorganisms, advances in molecular biology and genetic studies are now available to the environmental microbiologist. Our research has employed the use of microbiological culture media and biochemical tests in the identification of microbial populations in environmental samples. Also, different types of microscopic methods have been used in our studies. The trend now is on molecular approaches based on nucleic acid sequence analysis for direct measure of the abundance, diversity and phylogeny of microorganisms in the environment. This hereditary material (DNA or 16sRNA) is specific to species that can now be identified in a mixed population that is typical of environmental samples. Also the use of nucleic acid probes allows the determination of the taxonomic status of individual cells in complex assemblages in the ecosystem (Hurst, 1997). This method has the advantage that cells can be identified irrespective of their state of health. Thus, viable and nonculturable bacteria in the population can be included in the ecosystem. Moreover, there will then be little use of pure cultures that do not occur in most environmental samples.

Thus during my visit to Rutgers University, New Brunswick, USA in 2000, I worked in collaboration with Douglas Eveleigh using molecular methods to estimate the microbial biomass of an enclosed environment. Samples were taken from the alimentary tract of the giant African land snail, *Archachatina marginata* Swainson. Bacterial DNA in the samples was extracted for sequencing. The ability of gut bacteria to produce enzymes that breakdown components of snail feedstuff was also investigated. This was studied with a view to elucidating the roles of bacteria in digesting plant materials in snail gut ecosystem. Previous studies at the University of Lagos (Odiete & Akpata, 1983) revealed the presence of two undescribed or 'new' bacteria species namely; *Corynebacterium sp nov.* and *Flavobacterium sp nov.* The results are encouraging in the search of unusual environments for microbes with novel capabilities to meet the demands of industries.

Roles of Aquatic Microorganisms in Environmental Management

From the discussion it is clear that aquatic microbes impact on man and the environment in various ways and they play important roles in environmental management. Microbes are used for assessing the quality of water. For instance, if the count of heterotrophic bacteria is high it is a sign of organic matter in a water source, hence the water will be unsuitable for culinary purposes.

However there are many uses of water and the quality required depends on the use intended. Microbes are useful in prediction of impacts. The presence of *E. coli* indicates recent contamination of water with sewage or faeces with a high probability of the presence of pathogens in the water. Therefore it can be predicted that consumers of the water may suffer infection of the gastrointestinal tract. Isolation of *Clostridium perfringes* or enterococci indicates that the water had been contaminated at sometime. It is suggested that such water be studied to locate the source of pollution and necessary measures for abatement be taken immediately. In the abatement of pollution, standards are set of microbes that are monitored. Industries and organizations keep within the allowable limits or pay the penalty for non compliance. Treatment of industrial waste waters or domestic sewage is mandatory. A microcosm of microbes brings about the biodegradation of waste matter in the sewage treatment plant.

Unlike raw sewage, treated effluent is more amenable to the receiving environment on disposal. This shows that microbes are used in setting standards and in sewage treatment. Furthermore, the peculiar biodegradative abilities of some microbes have been employed in the rehabilitation of polluted environments. Some *Pseudomonas* species have been exploited in biological remediation of oil polluted environments because the bacteria can breakdown the crude oil.

Conclusion

Attention has been drawn to the fact that evolution of life started in the aquatic environment and microbes were the first formed living cells. To date some microbes remain in their original habitat of water which is abundant on the surface as well as in the aquifer on planet Earth. Microbes isolated from water and especially those in unusual or extreme habitats may have potentials that are novel and useful to man. Water is essential for sustainability of life. Unfortunately, the degradation of water quality is largely by human activities that impede the natural ability of autochthonous microbes to effect self-purification of water. Microorganisms are useful in sewage treatment and in water quality assessment. Knowledge of aquatic microbial ecology may be used in the control of water pollution. Environmental Impact Assessment (EIA) and maintenance of a healthy aquatic ecosystem would ensure sustainable development.

Recommendations

The responsibilities of a university professor may be grouped into three: Training of high level man power, carrying out research to generate new ideas and knowledge for sustainable development, and participation in the management of academic resources in terms of administration at different levels of the community.

It is customary at the end of an inaugural lecture to send feelers to the public on the relevance of the ivory tower research to national issues. In this lecture some of our research studies were discussed.

Under recommendations, I would like to highlight the limitations we face presently in the area of manpower development and also dwell on the need for community involvement in environmental management.

1. Manpower development involves human capacity building. The urriculum for Microbiology at the University of Lagos contains the essential elements required to meet the demands of environmental microbiologists anywhere. However, our students need to be familiar with some newer techniques. They will benefit more from the molecular approach so that they can be more marketable. Unfortunately, it is becoming increasingly difficult to organize enough laboratory practicals to support theory. Even the traditional methods lack space and consumable materials! The University of Lagos was not always like this!! There are too many students for the available spaces, and funds are inadequate for routine laboratory work. The recommendation is that more spaces be provided for practical work so as to enhance our understanding and practice of Microbiology.
2. Environmental Education. The elevation of the Federal Environmental Protection Agency to Federal Ministry of Environment is in line with global trends. Nigeria is playing a leadership role in environmental matters in Africa. Indeed the country is represented at international meetings on the Environment. However, this top administrative posture must be matched with grass-root knowledge and participation in environmental management. Individuals should recognize early signs of environmental degradation and know those to whom a report would receive quick response. Environmental issues are largely what are seen rather than what is said or written! In other words, emphasis should be on implementation of policies. Our leadership status should be reflected in the level of cleanliness and health of the ecosystem. To achieve this, Environmental Education must be implemented in the curricula of primary and secondary schools. This would infuse environmental awareness into our value system such that environmental consciousness becomes a national culture and a clean environment the pride of all Nigerians.

Aquatic Microbes Shape our World

The Earth is a complex and ever-changing combination of land, air, water and living organisms. These components are intricately linked so that processes occurring in one affect the others. Microbes play vital roles in this global system by driving biogeochemical cycles that affect the climate and move elements around the planet, making them available to other organisms. Without microbes, the Earth would be uninhabitable and yet they are the least understood life-forms on our planet.

The Marine and Freshwater Microbial Biodiversity programme has investigated how aquatic microbes shape the global system. Marine microbes play a critical role in regulating natural and man-made gases that affect climate. New research has let us cultivate previously-unknown bacteria that break down methybromide - a chemical that destroys stratospheric ozone. Scientists have investigated microbial methane production, and how marine viruses affect levels of dimethyl sulphide, a gas that promotes cloud formation. Other groups have studied how bacteria fix gaseous nitrogen for growth in seawater, and how they interact with trace metals in freshwater sediments, contaminated estuaries and coastal seas. Methyl bromide gas destroys a massive 25% of ozone lost from the stratosphere. It is released when biomass burns, when cars use leaded petrol, and some countries use it to fumigate soils and harvested crops. Researchers at the University of Warwick and the Plymouth Marine Laboratory have cultivated three new types of bacteria with enzymes that break down the gas. Using molecular probes, they discovered that marine environments harbour many different bacteria with this enzyme.

Methane is increasing in the atmosphere faster than carbon dioxide, and has 21 times its global warming potential. Methane is produced by archaea in the absence of oxygen, and researchers usually assume most of it comes from freshwater environments like wetlands and marshes. Scientists from Cardiff University used tracer and stable isotope techniques to study methane production at 21 sites, ranging from full freshwater to seawater. The team's results will help identify methane sources – a critical step towards reducing inputs to the atmosphere.

Marine micro-organisms also produce beneficial gases, for example dimethyl sulphide (DMS), the dominant sulphur trace gas in seawater. In laboratory culture and field mesocosm studies, researchers at the Marine Biological Association and the University of East Anglia showed that when viruses kill the marine phytoplankton *Emiliania huxleyi*, DMS production increases. DMS emitted from the sea is important in the global sulphur cycle. It also influences global climate by producing sulphate particles that can promote cloud formation, and hence altering how much of the Sun's energy the Earth reflects back to space.

Microbes can convert nitrogen gas to ammonia and organic nitrogen compounds – a critical process in the global nitrogen cycle. Levels of available nitrogen limit phytoplankton growth in the sea, yet more phytoplankton grow in some tropical and sub-tropical regions than known nitrogen inputs can support. Researchers from the Universities of Stirling and Newcastle used molecular methods to show that as-yet-uncultured nitrogen-fixing bacteria are widely distributed. Scientists used to think that microrganisms only fix nitrogen when they have to, because the process uses a lot of energy and other resources such as iron. So it was surprising to discover that key nitrogen-fixation genes in these bacteria were still operating when ammonia and nitrate were available in the seawater.

Living organisms need trace metals for various processes, but elevated levels can be toxic. Researchers from the Plymouth Marine Laboratory and the University of Southampton looked at how copper and zinc affected the bacterial assemblage, and the size and shape of aggregates (decaying phytoplankton debris and bacteria) in water from clean and metal-contaminated estuaries. They also used micro-electrodes to map oxygen concentration in marine aggregates. Scientists from the University of Lancaster developed a 2D imaging technique to assess how microbes influence geochemical processes in sediments. These projects help show how bacterial activity affects the mobility of trace metals at micro scales.

Chapter

10

Industrial Aspects of Amylase Enzymes

History of Enzymes

The history of modern enzyme technology really began in 1874 when the Danish chemist Christian Hansen produced the first specimen of rennet by extracting dried calves' stomachs with saline solution. Apparently this was the first enzyme preparation of relatively high purity used for industrial purposes.

This significant event had been preceded by a lengthy evolution. Enzymes have been used by man throughout the ages, either in the form of vegetables rich in enzymes, or in the form of microorganisms used for a variety of purposes, for instance in brewing processes, in baking, and in the production of alcohol. It is generally known that enzymes were already used in the production of cheese since old times.

Even though the action of enzymes has been recognised and enzymes have been used throughout history, it was quite recently that their importance were realised. Enzymatic processes, particularly fermentation, were the focus of numerous studies in the 19th century and many valuable discoveries in this field were made. A particularly important experiment was the isolation of the enzyme complex from malt by Payen and Persoz in 1833. This extract, like malt itself, converts gelatinised starch into sugars, primarily into maltose, and was termed 'diastase'.

Development progressed during the following decades, particularly in the field of fermentation where the achievements by Schwann, Liebig, Pasteur and Kuhne were of the greatest importance. The dispute between Liebig and Pasteur concerning the fermentation process caused much heated debate. Liebig claimed that fermentation resulted from chemical process and that yeast was a non-viable substance continuously in the process of breaking down. Pasteur, on the other hand, argued that fermentation did not occur unless viable organisms were present.

The dispute was finally settled in 1897, after the death of both adversaries, when the Buchner brothers demonstrated that cell free yeast extract could convert glucose into ethanol and carbon dioxide just like viable yeast cells. In other words, the conversion was not ascribable to yeast cells as such, but to their non-viable enzymes.

In 1876, William Kuhne proposed that the name 'enzyme' be used as the new term to denote phenomena previously known as 'unorganised ferments', that is, ferments isolated from the viable organisms in which they were formed. The word itself means 'in yeast' and is derived from the Greek 'en' meaning 'in', and 'zyme' meaning 'yeast' or 'leaven'.

Early Developments in Japan

During the early part of this century, enzyme technology was also developing slowly but surely outside Europe. In the Far East, an age-old tradition prevailed where mould fungi, the so-called koji, were (and still are) used in the production of certain foodstuffs and flavour additives based on soya protein (shoyu, miso, tempeh) and fermented beverages (sake, alcohol). Koji is prepared from steamed rice into which a mixture of mould fungi is inoculated, the composition of the mixture being passed down from generation to generation. This formed the basis which the Japanese scientist Takamine developed a fermentation process for the industrial production of fungal amylase; the process included the culture of Aspergillus oryzae on moist rice or wheat bran. The product was called 'Takadiastase' and it is still used as a digestive aid. The method of fermentation suggested by Takamine, the 'surface culture' or 'semi-solid culture' is still actively used in the production of various enzymes.

Textile Desizing

At about the same time as Takamine was developing his novel fermentation technique, another field was being opened up for the use of enzymes-the desizing of textiles. Previously, textiles were treated with acid, alkali or oxidising agents, or soaked in water for several days so that naturally occurring microorganisms could break down the starch. However, both of these methods were difficult to control and sometimes damaged or discoloured the material. It represented great progress, therefore, when crude enzyme extracts in the form of malt extract, or later, in the form of pancreas extract, were first used to carry out desizing.

Bacterial amylase derived from Bacillus subtilis was used for desizing, the first time by Boidin and Effront as early as 1917.

Leather Bating

Investigations carried out by the German chemist and industrial magnate Otto Rohm before World War I were of great importance for the further development of the industrial use of enzymes. Among other things, he studied the so called 'bating' process, a step in the preparation of hides and skins prior to tanning.

According to tradition, bating required the excrement of dogs and pigeons, a fact that did not improve the image of tanning which was considered a stinking and unpleasant activity. Rohm's theory was that these excrements exerted their effect because they contained residual amounts of the animals' digestive enzymes. If this was so, it might be possible to use extracts of the pancreas directly for bating. Such extracts were tried and produced the expected positive results. Naturally, Rohm accepted this as confirmation of the correctness of his theory, but later experiments showed that it was not the animals' enzymes that were active, but rather enzymes of bacteria growing in the intestinal tract.

The First Detergent Enzyme

Parallel to his studies of the problems involved in tanning, Rohm investigated other processes where enzymes would prove even more valuable. Nevertheless, his efforts were not to score a success until 50 years later. Rohm actually developed the first method for washing protein stained cloth in detergents containing enzymes and manufactured the first detergent preparation containing enzymes.

The enzyme preparation used was pancreatin (extracted from pancreatic glands), which contains the protein degrading enzyme trypsin. Breakthrough in detergents was made in 1959, when a Swiss chemist Dr. Jaag, developed a new product called Bio 40 containing a bacterial protease instead of trypsin.

Sugars from Starch

A very important field in which enzymes have proved to be of great value over the last 15-20 years is the starch industry. In 1950s, fungal amylase was used in the manufacture of specific types of syrup, i.e., those containing a range of sugars, which could not be produced by conventional acid hydrolysis. The real turning point was reached early in the 1960s when an enzyme glucoamylase, was launched for the first time, which could completely break down starch into glucose. Within a few years, almost all glucose production was re-organised and enzyme hydrolysis was used instead of acid hydrolysis because of the more benefits such as greater yield, higher degree of purity and easier crystallisation.

The process was further improved by the introduction of a new technique used for the enzymatic pre-treatment (liquefaction) of starch by using a heat-stable alpha amylase.

Years of research in biochemistry and biotechnology have boosted knowledge of enzymes for industries as well as research. Many new techniques have been established to modify enzymes or increase their yields. New techniques for purification of enzymes are constantly developing and so are being discovered new application of enzymes in medicine, research and industries.

Enzymes for Textile

At Maps, we continuously develop our product line in order to have innovative enzymes with unique performance features for existing and new applications within the textile industry. Our R&D aims to provide innovative products for fabric treatment reducing process time, chemical consumption and energy costs in compliance with sustainable development. We provide a range of enzymes like amylases, cellulases, catalase, pectinase and protease for various textile wet-processing applications like desizing, bio-polishing, denim finishing, bleach clean-up, bio-scouring and de-wooling.

Desizing

For fabrics made from cotton or blends, the warp threads are coated with an adhesive substance know as 'size'; to prevent the threads breaking during weaving. Although many different compounds have been used to size fabrics, starch and its derivatives have been the most common sizing agent. After weaving, the size must be removed again in order to prepare the fabric for dyeing and finishing.

This process (desizing) must be carried out by treating the fabric with chemicals such as acids, alkali or oxidising agents. However starch-breaking enzymes (amylases) are preferred for desizing due to their high efficiency and specific action. Amylases bring about complete removal of the size without any harmful effects on the fabric. Another benefit of enzymes compared to strong chemicals mentioned above is that enzymes are environment friendly.

Maps offers a range of amylases for desizing which work at different temperatures and for different equipments.

Palkozyme	Alpha amylase for low-medium temperature conventional desizing.
Palkozyme Ultra	Alpha amylase for low-medium temperature desizing
Palkozyme Plus	Alpha amylase for high temperature desizing
Palkozyme HT	Heat-stable alpha amylase for high temperature desizing
Palkozyme CLX	Alpha amylase for low temperature desizing

Bio-Polishing

Cotton and other natural fibres based on cellulose can be improved by an enzymatic treatment known as Bio-Polishing. This treatment gives the fabric a smoother and glossier appearance. The treatment is used to remove 'fuzz'-the tiny strands of fibre that protrude from the surface of yarn. A ball of fuzz is called a 'pill' in the textile trade. After Bio-Polishing, the fuzz and pilling are reduced. The other benefits of removing fuzz are a softer and smoother handle, and superior colour brightness.

Maps offers a range of cellulases for bio-polishing which work on depending on fibre, fabric type and equipments.

Palkofeel	Cellulase for bio-polishing cotton and blended fabric and garment
Palkofeel C	Cellulase for bio-polishing cotton fabric and garments
Palkosoft	Cellulase for bio-polishing cotton and blended fabric and garment

Denim Finishing

Many garments are subjected to a wash treatment to give them a slightly worn look; example is the stonewashing of denim jeans. In the traditional stonewashing process, the blue denim was faded by the abrasive action of pumice stones on the garment surface. Nowadays, denim finishers are using a special cellulase.

Cellulase works by loosening the indigo dye on the denim in a process know as 'Bio-Stonewashing'. A small dose of enzyme can replace several kilograms of pumice stones. The use of less pumice stones results in less damage to garment, machine and less pumice dust in the laundry environment. Bio-Stonewashing has opened up new possibilities in denim finishing by increasing the variety of finishes available. For example, it is now possible to fade denim to a greater degree without running the risk of damaging the garment. Productivity can also be increased because laundry machines contain fewer stones or no stones and more garments.

Maps offers a range of cellulases for denim finishing, each with its own special properties. These can be used either alone or in combination with pumice stones in order to obtain a specific look.

Palkowash	Cellulase for bio-stonewashing denims used in garment wet-processing
Palkostone	Cellulase for bio-stonewashing denims used in garment wet-processing
Palkocel	Cellulase for bio-stonewashing denims used in garment wet-processing

Bleach Clean-up

Natural fabrics such as cotton are normally bleached with hydrogen peroxide before dyeing. Bleaches are highly reactive chemicals and any peroxide left on the fabric can interfere with the dyeing process. A thorough 'Bleach Cleanup' is necessary. The traditional method is to neutralize the bleach with a reducing agent, but the dose has to be controlled precisely. Enzymes present a more convenient alternative because they are easier and quicker to use. A small dose of catalase is capable of breaking down hydrogen peroxide into water and oxygen. Compared with the traditional clean-up methods, the enzymatic process results in cleaner waste water or reduced water consumption.

Maps offer catalase for removing residual hydrogen peroxide after the bleaching of cotton. It reduces the rinsing necessary to remove bleach or it can be used to replace chemical treatments.

Palkoperox	Catalase for bleach clean-up i.e. removal residual hydrogen peroxide after the bleaching of cotton.

Bio-Scouring

Cotton yarn or fabric, prior to dyeing or printing, goes through a number of processes in a textile processing unit. A very important process is scouring. In this process, non-cellulosic components from native cotton are completely or partially removed. Scouring gives a fabric with a high and even wet ability so that it can be bleached and dyed successfully. Today, highly alkaline chemicals caustic soda are used for scouring. These chemicals not only remove the non-cellulosic impurities from the cotton, but also attack the cellulose leading to heavy strength loss and weight loss in the fabric. Furthermore, using these hazardous chemicals result in high COD (chemical oxygen demand), BOD (biological oxygen demand) and TDS, in the waste water.

Recently a new enzymatic scouring process know as 'Bio-Scouring' is used in textile wet-processing with which all non-cellulosic components from native cotton are completely or partially removed. After this Bio-Scouring process, the cotton has an intact cellulose structure, with lower weight loss and strength loss. The fabric gives better wetting and penetration properties, making subsequent bleach process easy and resultantly giving much better dye uptake.

Enzymes for Leather

One of the oldest applications of industrial enzymes is processing hides and skins for leather. Hides and skins contain proteins and fat in between collagen fibres and before tanning; these substances should be partially and fully removed. The proteins can be removed by proteases and lipases as well as other chemicals can remove the fat. Today, proteases and lipases are mainly used for soaking, bating and enzyme assisted un-hairing. Using lipases to dissolve and remove fat is a recent development and lipases are now extensively used for leather processing in many parts of the world.

Maps is a major supplier of enzyme to the leather industry in India and across the globe. We offer total enzyme solutions for bating, un-haring, degreasing and soaking in the beam-house processes. With the introduction of our new range of products based on Microorganisms, we assure to provide clean and green leather tanneries.

Bating

To make leather pliable, the hides and skins require an enzymatic treatment before tanning know as bating. During bating, scud is loosened and other unwanted proteins are removed. Bating de-swells swollen pelts and prepares leather for tanning. It makes the grain surface of the finished leather clean, smooth and fine. Bating with enzymes is an indispensable operation of leather processing to obtain best quality of leather and cannot be substituted with a chemical process. Traditional methods for bating employed manure of dog, pigeon or hen. These were very unpleasant, unreliable and slow methods. Bio-technical developments in science have now completely replaced these methods with use of industrial enzymes.

Maps offers a range of proteases for bating which work in different pH conditions.

Palkobate	Protease for bating in alkaline pH conditions
Palkocid	Protease for bating in acidic pH conditions

Soaking

Soaking is first important operation of leather processing. Hides and skins received into a tannery are in the four conditions, as green or fresh, as wet salted, as dry salted or as dried. It is advisable to carry out soaking for all types of skin and hides to obtain best quality leather. Soaking cleans hides and skins by removing dirt, blood, flesh, grease, dung etc. and most importantly, re-hydrates them to bring skins as far as possible back to state of green hides. Soaking agents fall into three categories, like Chemical Agents, Surface-active agents and Enzymatic agents. Enzymatic agents are biocatalyst. Specific protease and lipase enzymes enhance water uptake by dissolving intrafibrillary proteins that cement fibres together and disperse fats and oils together with dirt and other contaminants present on skin.

Maps offers a range of protease and lipase for soaking which work in different pH conditions.

Palkosoak	A mixture of protease and lipase for soaking in alkaline pH conditions
Palkosoak ACP	A mixture of protease and lipase for soaking in acidic pH conditions

Un-hairing

The conventional and most wide spread way to remove hair from bovine hides is to use lime and sodium sulphide in a hair-burning process. They dissolve the hair and open up the fibre structure. Most importantly, enzyme-assisted un-hairing results in a cleaner grain surface and improved area yield and softness. The use of a specific protease also offers tanneries a number of options. For instance, the sulphide and lime requirements can be reduced by as much as 40% while maintaining the same liming time. Alternatively tanners can shorten the liming time by at least half without any loss of quality.

Another possibility is to avoid the use of amines, which can be converted into carcinogenic compounds. The hair-burning process is the most widespread but a better alternative to this, is the hair-saving process, which is environment friendly, where the hair is not dissolved but can be filtered out from the liming float. It is possible to reduce the COD up to 50% and BOD up to 30% in waste discharges.

Maps offers a specific protease for un-hairing which can be used either alone or in combination lime and sodium sulphide:

Palkodehair	Protease for un-hairing in high alkaline pH conditions

Degreasing

Lipases are a type of enzyme that specifically degrades fat and so cannot damage the leather itself. Lipases hydrolyse not just the fat on the outside of the hides and skins, but also the fat inside the skin structure. Once most of the natural fat has been removed, subsequent chemical treatments such as tanning, re-tanning and dyeing have a better effect.

The main advantages of using lipases are a more uniform colour and a cleaner appearance. Lipases also improve the production of hydrophobic (waterproof) leather; makers of leather for car upholstery have commented that 'fogging' is reduced. This is the term for the build-up of a film of chemicals on the inside of car windscreens. Lipases represent a more environmentally sound method of removing fat. For bovine hides, lipases allow tensides to be replaced completely. For sheepskins, which contain up to 40% fat, the use of solvents is very common and these can also be replaced with lipases and surfactants. Solvents tend to dry out the skin and give it a pale colour.

If surfactants are used for sheepskins, they are usually not as effective and may be harmful to the environment. Stronger surfactants such as nonyl phenol ethoxylate have a better effect but they are more detrimental to the environment. When using lipases, the original surfactant dosage can be reduced by at least 50% in the case of both sheepskins and pigskins. In addition, nonyl phenol ethoxylate can be substituted with more biodegradable surfactants.

Enzymes for Baking

As a result of our R&D over the past few years, today Maps has a versatile product range of enzymes for the baking industry. Apart from individual enzymes like amylase, xylanase, protease, cellulase, we also have a range of tailored enzyme cocktails (mixtures of different enzymes) to solve problems in certain baking applications. Our customers for our baking enzymes are the baking improver industry or the milling industry, the Wafer, Biscuit and Cracker industry, etc.

Like all other living material, the cells in cereal grains used for flour contain enzymes. The most important enzymes in flour are the amylases and proteases. However, the quantities of these enzymes are not always ideal for baking purposes and supplementary enzymes often need to be added.

Bread-making

Bread is the most common and traditional foods around the world. But bread actually has close links with enzymes. For years, enzymes such as malt and fungal alpha-amylase have been used in bread making. Due to the changes in the baking industry and the ever-increasing demand for more natural products, enzymes have gained real importance in bread-making.

The dough for bread, rolls, buns, etc. consists of flour, water, yeast, salt and other ingredients such as sugar and fat. Flour consists of gluten, starch, non-starch polysaccharides, lipids, etc. When the dough is made, the yeast starts to work on the fermentable sugars, transforming them into alcohol and carbon dioxide, thus rising the dough.

In the beginning, the fermentation goes smoothly whether sugar has been added or not, because flour always contains a certain amount of fermentable sugar. But when this has been used up, the fermentation process will cease unless new supplies of sugar are made available to the yeast.

Amylases degrade starch and produce small dextrins for the yeast to act. Gluten is a combination of proteins, which form a large network during dough formation. This network holds the gas in dough proofing and baking. The strength of this network is very important for the quality of all bread raised by yeast. Enzymes such as proteases, xylanases and lipases directly or indirectly improve the strength of the gluten network and so improve the quality the bread.

Dough Improvement

A small percentage of pentosans (non-starch polysaccharides) are present in flour. Pentosans have an important role in bread quality due to their water absorption capability and interaction with gluten, which is vital for the formation of the loaf structure. By hydrolysing the pentosans using some enzymes like hemicellulase, pentosanase or xylanase, the dough becomes easier to handle and the resulting bread has a bigger loaf volume and an improved crumb structure

Maps offers a range of amylases, proteases and xylanases for bread-making and dough improvement

Palkoamylo	Fungal alpha amylase
Palkobake X	Fungal xylanase
Palkotase ACP	Fungal protease

Flour Supplementation

Alpha amylases have significant effects on baked goods. If the content is low, this leads to low dextrin production and poor gas production. This in turn results in inferior quality bread with reduced size and poor crust colour.

To compensate for the deficiencies of the grain, it is necessary to add either sugar or alpha amylase. The addition of enzymes offers certain advantages over sugar. At a flour mill, it is possible to standardize the enzyme content of the flour so that a uniform commodity can be supplied. Furthermore, enzymes bring about a gradual formation of sugar, which matches the needs of the yeast. When the dough is placed in the oven, the steadily increasing temperature leads to an increase in the enzymes' rate of reaction and more sugar is produced. Malt flour and malt extract can be used as enzyme supplements as malt is rich in alpha amylases. However, it is better to use a fungal alpha amylase.

The alpha-amylases degrade the damaged starch in wheat flour into small dextrins, thus allowing yeast to work continuously during dough fermentation, proofing and the early stage of baking. This result in improved bread volume and crumb texture. In addition, the small oligosaccharides and sugars such as glucose and maltose produced by these enzymes enhance the reactions for the browning of the crust and baked flavour.

Maps offers a range of amylases and xylanases for flour supplementation, each with its own special properties which work to obtain specific needs of wheat flour.

Palkoflour	Fungal alpha amylase
Palkoamylo	Fungal alpha amylase
Palkoflour AX	A mixture of fungal alpha amylase and xylanase

Production of Biscuit and Crackers

Another application of enzymes in baking is in the production of biscuits and crackers. The requirements of the flour are altogether different from those in bread-making; a 'soft flour' which produces a dough with pronounced plastic properties is preferred. For this purpose, flour with relatively low protein content is desirable. The gluten protein structure should not be too strong, otherwise the dough will be too difficult to handle.

Unless flour with these properties is available, it is necessary to add an agent to weaken the gluten. Reducing agents (substances which have the opposite effect to oxidizing agents) have been used for this purpose, in particular sodium bisulphite. The bisulphite has the desired effect on the gluten, but unfortunately it affects other substances in the flour, including the content of vitamin B1 (thiamine). This vitamin is completely or partially destroyed. Sodium bisulphite has been banned in certain countries and is becoming less popular due to health risks.

An alternative is the application of a protein-degrading enzyme. This softens the gluten without affecting the other constituents of the dough. Several fungal and bacterial proteases can be used for this purpose. Proteases can also be used when making bread with 'hard flour' i.e. flour high in gluten protein.

Enzymes for Alcohol

The production of fermented alcoholic drinks from starch-based raw materials has been practised since long. The raw material for this differs from, maize (corn) and rye to barley and wheat for whisky and other cereals for grain spirits. But whatever the raw materials are, starch is still the basic ingredient. Starch is composed of long chains of glucose molecules and these have to be broken down into smaller molecules, which the yeast can transform into alcohol. Enzymes can carry out this process in two stages-liquefaction and saccharification.

Traditionally, enzymes have been provided by adding malt. However, since quite some time, there has been a change and in many countries malt has been totally replaced from distilling operations by the use of enzymes. There are a lot of advantages using industrial enzymes instead of malt, like small quantities of enzyme addition can replace large quantities of malt, resulting easy handling and storage. Even raw material costs are reduced by nearly 30% when switching to commercial enzymes.

Starch Liquefaction

Before enzymes can attack the starch, it must be gelatinised. This is usually done by pressure-cooking. Now-a-days, the old no pressure cooking method has been gaining in popularity, especially in smaller distilleries. Instead of temperatures around 150?C, the maximum temperature ranges from 60?C to 95?C. This results in energy savings and also capital savings since pressure vessels are not required. Whatever the processing technique, alpha amylases are used to break down the gelatinised starch to shorter molecules (dextrins).

Starch Saccharification

Saccharification is the second step in the process. A glucoamylase enzyme is used to break down the starch molecules and the dextrins. This enzyme is capable of achieving the complete degradation of the starch to fermentable sugars (glucose). During fermentation, these sugars are converted into alcohol by yeast in simultaneous saccharification and fermentation process.

Fermentation Improvement

Cereals, particularly maize have low soluble nitrogen. This results in poor yeast growth and longer fermentation time. By adding a small amount of protease enzyme helps in yeast growth and reduce fermentation time. During distillation process it may be necessary to reduce viscosity of the fermentation broth. To facilitate this beta glucanase/pentosanase enzymes are added.

Enzymes for Brewing

Traditionally production of beer is by mixing crushed barley malt and hot water in large vessel known as mash copper. This process is known as 'mashing'. Apart from malt, other starch-based cereals such as maize (corn), sorghum, rice and barley, or pure starch itself, are added to the mash. These are known as adjuncts. After mashing, the mash is filtered in a lauter tun and the liquid, known as 'sweet wort', is then run off to the copper, where it is boiled with hops. The 'hopped wort' is cooled and transferred to the fermentation vessels where yeast is added. After the fermentation, the so-called 'green beer' is matured before the final filtration and bottling.

Liquefying Adjuncts

Adjuncts are used as an extra source of starch in brewing and usually consist of cereals. Protein also plays a vital role in fermentation by providing soluble nitrogen compounds that the yeast needs. Since the protein proportion in some types of adjunct is very small, it may be necessary to provide extra protein in the wort. This can be done by utilising the protein in the malt more efficiently. By adding a protein splitting (protease) enzyme, more protein can be solubilised and made available to the yeast. In their natural form, starch-based cereals such as maize grits and rice are boiled before being added to the malt mash. The boiled (gelatinised) cereals are very viscous and need to be thinned (liquefied) before they can be pumped into the mash copper. This is done using an alpha amylase. Heat-stable alpha amylases are also available that are effective even at 100?C to ensure full liquefaction of the starch.

Filtration

Slow rate of filtration is generally a problem when the mash is run off in the lauter tun and also during the final filtration of the beer. This is due to the presence of certain polysaccharides, mainly beta-glucans and pentosans, which are found in barley and poorly modified barley malt. The solution is to break down the beta-glucans using a beta-glucanase added during mashing or at the start of the fermentation process.

Enzymes for Detergent

For most people, the most popular known application of enzymes is in the manufacture of enzymatic washing agents (detergents). Since last 40 years, the use of enzymes in detergents has been the largest of all enzyme applications. Consumers of detergents are actual users of an enzymatic product. In majority of other applications, enzymes are used as auxiliary agents at some point in the manufacturing process and are not, as a rule, present in the finished product-not at any rate in an active form.

Proteases

Proteases are the most widely used enzymes in the detergent industry. They remove protein stains such as grass, blood, egg and human sweat. These organic stains have a tendency to adhere strongly to textile fibres. The proteins act as glues, preventing the water-borne detergent systems from removing some of the other components of the soiling, such as pigments and street dirt. The inefficiency of non-enzymatic detergents at removing proteins can result in permanent stains due to oxidation and denaturing caused by bleaching and drying. Blood, for example, will leave a rust-coloured spot unless it is removed before bleaching. Proteases hydrolyse proteins and break them down into more soluble polypeptides or free amino acids. As a result of the combined effect of surfactants and enzymes, stubborn stains can be removed from fibres.

Lipases

Though enzymes can easily digest protein stains, oily and fatty stains have always been troublesome to remove. The trend towards lower washing temperatures has made the removal of grease spots an even bigger problem. This applies particularly to materials made up of a blend of cotton and polyester. The lipase is capable of removing fatty stains such as fats, butter, salad oil, sauces and the tough stains on collars and cuffs.

Amylases

Amylases are used to remove residues of starch-based foods like potatoes, spaghetti, custards, gravies and chocolate. This type of enzyme can be used in laundry detergents as well as in dishwashing detergents.

Cellulases

The development of detergent enzymes has mainly focused on enzymes capable of removing stains. However, a cellulase enzyme has properties enabling it to modify the structure of cellulose fibre on cotton and cotton blends. When it is added to a detergent, it results into the following effects: Colour brightening-When garments made of cotton or cotton blends have been washed several times, they tend to get a 'fluffy' look and the colours become duller. This effect is due to the formation of microfibrils that become partly detached from the main fibres. The light falling on the garment is reflected back to a greater extent giving the impression that the colour is duller. These fibrils, however, can be degraded by the cellulase enzyme, restoring a smooth surface to the fibre and restoring the garment to its original colour. Softening-The enzyme also has a significant softening effect on the fabric, probably due to the removal of the microfibrils. Soil removal-Some dirt particles are trapped in the network of microfibrils and are released when the microfibrils are removed by the cellulase enzyme.

Enzymes for Starch

In the early 19th century, it was discovered that by boiling starch with acid it could be converted into a sweet-tasting substance, which consisted mainly of glucose. Since then acids have been used widely for breaking down starch into glucose. This technique does have a number of drawbacks. The DE (dextrose equivalent) value is used as an indication of the degree of hydrolysis of syrup. The DE value of starch is zero and that of dextrose is 100. In the last 25 years, as new enzymes are available, starch hydrolysis technology has move away from acids to enzymes. Enzymatic starch conversion, depending on the enzymes used, syrups with different compositions and physical properties of starch. There are three basic steps in enzymatic starch conversion: liquefaction, saccharification and isomerisation.

Starch Liquefaction

Firstly, there is a liquefaction process. A starch suspension containing 30-40% dry matter is first gelatinised and liquefied. By using heat-stable bacterial alpha amylase, 'maltodextrin' is obtained which contains mainly different oligosaccharides and dextrins. Maltodextrins are only slightly sweet and they usually undergo further conversion. In most starch conversion plants, starch liquefaction takes place in a jet-cooking process. The heat stable alpha amylase is added to the starch slurry after pH adjustment, and the slurry is pumped through a jet cooker. Live steam is injected here to raise the temperature to 105°C, and the slurry is then passed through a series of holding tubes for 5-7 minutes, which is necessary to gelatinise the starch fully. Then the temperature of the partially liquefied starch is reduced to 90-100°C by flashing, and the enzyme is allowed to react further at this temperature for 1-2 hours until the required DE (Dextrose Equivalent) is obtained.

Starch Saccharification

Saccharification is the second step in the process. Depending of the desired end product, a glucoamylase or a fungal alpha amylase is used further break down the Maltodextrins. The glucoamylase can hydrolyse starch completely to glucose along with, a little maltose and isomaltose. A pullulanase is a de-branching enzyme that can also be used to aid saccharification. Fungal alpha amylases can also be added in order to produce syrups with a higher maltose content, which means high fermentability and a relatively high degree of sweetness.

Isomerisation

Further going one step ahead, a proportion of the glucose can be isomerised into fructose, which is about twice as sweet as glucose. An immobilized glucose isomerase is used.

Enzymes for Animal Feed

Animal feed is composed of plant material, cereals and vegetable proteins, which cannot be fully digested and utilised by animals. However, feed utilization and digestion can often be increased by the addition of external enzymes to the feed. Many cereals have a proportion of their energy in the form of non-starch polysaccharides (NSPs), more commonly known as fibre. Enzymes are to break down these NSPs, which lead in increase of metabolisable energy and protein utilisation.

In some cereals, a large part of the NSP is soluble and causes high viscosity in the small intestine of a monogastric animal. As a result, digestion becomes impaired. Selected microbial enzymes can partially degrade this NSP, lowering viscosity in the intestine and improving feed utilisation. Many vegetable protein sources, such as soybean meal, also contain NSP. The addition of selected microbial enzymes can be used to break down the NSP and make it available to the animal. Just as with cereals, the metabolisable energy and protein utilisation for vegetable protein sources can be improved by using the correct combination of amylases and proteases.

In almost all plant material used for animal feed, a large part of the mineral phosphorus is bound in the form of phytic acid, which cannot be degraded by monogastric animals. Phytase liberates part of the bound phosphorus and makes it possible to reduce the phosphorus content of the feed by 25-30%. The R & D centre at Maps has successful produced phytase, and soon shall be commercially launched.

Enzyme for Poultry Feed

The main cost in the raising of poultry is the feed, which is mainly cereal-based. Maize (corn) has a low content of soluble NSPs and is considered to be an ideal cereal. Other cereals contain higher amounts of NSPs that normally impair feed utilisation. It is possible to partially degrading these NSPs with selected enzymes acting on specific raw materials. For example, when using a standard dose of the Maps xylanase enzymes for poultry feed, the metabolisable energy value for wheat increases.

Some cereals are also avoided in poultry diets due to the adverse effects caused by NSP. Barley is a prime example because inclusion of more than 10% barley in broiler diets gives rise to wet and sticky droppings as well as reduced growth rates. This is due to beta glucan, a soluble, high viscosity NSP located in the cell walls of the barley grain. By adding microbial enzymes to the barley based feed, the NSP could be degraded giving an improvement in droppings, better feed utilisation and faster growth rate.

How are Enzymes Made?

The starting point for enzyme production is a vial of a selected strain of microorganisms. They will be nurtured and fed until they multiply many thousand times. Then the desired end-product is recovered from the fermentation broth and sold as a standardised product. A single bacteria or fungus is able to produce only a very small portion of the enzyme, but billions microorganisms, however, can produce large amounts of enzyme. The process of multiplying microorganisms by millions is called fermentation. Fermentation to produce industrial enzymes starts with a vial of dried or frozen microorganisms called a production strain. One very important aspect of fermentation is sterilisation. In order to cultivate a particular production strain, it is first necessary to eliminate all the native microorganisms present in the raw materials and equipment. If proper sterilisation is not done, other wild organisms will quickly outnumber the production strain and no production will occur.

The production strain is first cultivated in a small flask containing nutrients. The flask is placed in an incubator, which provides the optimal temperature for the microorganism cells to germinate. Once the flask is ready, the cells are transferred to a seed fermenter, which is a large tank containing previously sterilised raw materials and water known as the medium. Seed fermentation allows the cells to reproduce and adapt to the environment and nutrients that will be encountered later on. After the seed fermentation, the cells are transferred to a larger tank, the main fermenter, where fermentation time, temperature, pH and air are controlled to optimise growth. When this fermentation is complete, the mixture of cells, nutrients and enzymes, called the broth, is ready for filtration and purification.

Filtration and purification termed as downstream processing is done after enzyme fermentation. The enzymes are extracted from the fermentation broth by various chemical treatments to ensure efficient extraction, followed by removal of the broth using either centrifugation or filtration. Followed by a series of other filtration processes, the enzymes are finally separated from the water using an evaporation process. After this the enzymes are formulated and standardised in form of powder, liquid or granules.

Chapter

11

Biological Warfare: A Serious Threat in the 21st Century

Characteristics of Biological Weapons

Anti-personnel

Ideal characteristics of a biological agent to be used as a weapon against humans are high infectivity, high virulence, non-availability of vaccines, and availability of an effective and efficient delivery system. Stability of the weaponized agent (ability of the agent to retain its infectivity and virulence after a prolonged period of storage) may also be desirable, particularly for military applications.

The primary difficulty is not the production of the biological agent, as many biological agents used in weapons can often be manufactured relatively quickly, cheaply and easily. Rather, it is the weaponization, storage and delivery in an effective vehicle to a vulnerable target that pose significant problems.

For example, *Bacillus anthracis* is considered an effective agent for several reasons. First, it forms hardy spores, perfect for dispersal aerosols. Second, this organism is not considered transmissible from person to person, and thus rarely if ever causes secondary infections. A pulmonary anthrax infection starts with ordinary influenza-like symptoms and progresses to a lethal hemorrhagic mediastinitis within 3–7 days, with a fatality rate that is 90% or higher in untreated patients. Finally, friendly personnel can be protected with suitable antibiotics. A large-scale attack using anthrax would require the creation of aerosol particles of 1.5 to 5 microns. Too large and the particles would not reach the lower respiratory tract. Too small and the particles would be exhaled back out into the atmosphere.

At this size, conductive powders tend to aggregate because of electrostatic charges, hindering dispersion. So the material must be treated to insulate and neutralize the charges. The weaponized agent must be resistant to degradation by rain and ultraviolet radiation from sunlight, while retaining the ability to efficiently infect the human lung. There are other technological difficulties as well, chiefly relating to storage of the weaponized agent.

Agents considered for weaponization, or known to be weaponized, include bacteria such as *Bacillus anthracis*, *Brucella spp.*, *Burkholderia mallei*, *Burkholderia pseudomallei*, *Chlamydophila psittaci*, *Coxiella burnetii*, *Francisella tularensis*, some of the Rickettsiaceae (especially *Rickettsia prowazekii* and *Rickettsia rickettsii*), *Shigella spp.*, *Vibrio cholerae*, and *Yersinia pestis*. Many viral agents have been studied and/or weaponized, including some of the Bunyaviridae (especially Rift Valley fever virus), Ebolavirus, many of the Flaviviridae (especially Japanese encephalitis virus), Machupo virus, Marburg virus, Variola virus, and Yellow fever virus. Fungal agents that have been studied include *Coccidioides spp.*.

Toxins that can be used as weapons include ricin, staphylococcal enterotoxin B, botulinum toxin, saxitoxin, and many mycotoxins. These toxins and the organisms that produce them are sometimes referred to as select agents. In the United States, their possession, use, and transfer are regulated by the Centres for Disease Control and Prevention's Select Agent Program.

Anti-agriculture

Biological warfare can also specifically target plants to destroy crops or defoliate vegetation. The United States and Britain discovered plant growth regulators (i.e., herbicides) during the Second World War, and initiated an herbicidal warfare program that was eventually used in Malaya and Vietnam in counter insurgency. Though herbicides are chemicals, they are often grouped with biological warfare as bioregulators in a similar manner as biotoxins. Scorched earth tactics or destroying livestock and farmland were carried out in the Vietnam war (cf. Agent Orange) and Eelam War in Sri Lanka.

The United States developed an anti-crop capability during the Cold War that used plant diseases (bioherbicides, or mycoherbicides) for destroying enemy agriculture. It was believed that destruction of enemy agriculture on a strategic scale could thwart Sino-Soviet aggression in a general war. Diseases such as wheat blast and rice blast were weaponized in aerial spray tanks and cluster bombs for delivery to enemy watersheds in agricultural regions to initiate epiphytotics (epidemics among plants). When the United States renounced its offensive biological warfare program in 1969 and 1970, the vast majority of its biological arsenal was composed of these plant diseases.

In 1980s Soviet Ministry of Agriculture had successfully developed variants of foot-and-mouth disease, and rinderpest against cows, African swine fever for pigs, and psittacosis to kill chicken. These agents were prepared to spray them down from tanks attached to airplanes over hundreds of miles. The secret program was code-named "Ecology". Attacking animals is another area of biological warfare intended to eliminate animal resources for transportation and food. In the First World War, German agents were arrested attempting to inoculate draft animals with anthrax, and they were believed to be responsible for outbreaks of glanders in horses and mules. The British tainted small feed cakes with anthrax in the Second World War as a potential means of attacking German cattle for food denial, but never employed the weapon. In the 1950s, the United States had a field trial with hog cholera. During the Mau Mau Uprising in 1952, the poisonous latex of the African milk bush was used to kill cattle.

Unconnected with inter-human wars, humans have deliberately introduced the rabbit disease Myxomatosis, originating in South America, to Australia and Europe, with the intention of reducing the rabbit population- which had devastating but temporary results, with wild rabbit populations reduced to a fraction of their former size but survivors developing immunity and increasing again.

Biodefence

Biodefence refers to short term, local, usually military measures to restore biosecurity to a given group of persons in a given area — in the civilian terminology, it is a very robust biohazard response. It is technically possible to apply biodefence measures to protect animals or plants, but this is generally uneconomic. However, protection of water supplies and food supplies are often a critical part of biodefence. Various definitions of biosafety emerged in different professions to guarantee non-human health. Biodefence is most often discussed in the context of biowar or bioterrorism, and is generally considered a military or emergency response term.

Biodefence applies to two distinct target populations: civilian non-combatant and military combatant (troops in the field).

Biodefence of Troops in the Field

The Department of Defence (or "DoD") has focused since at least 1998 on the development and application of vaccine-based biodefences. In a July 2001 report commissioned by the DoD, the "DoD-critical products" were stated as vaccines against anthrax (AVA and Next Generation), smallpox, plague, tularemia, botulinum, ricin, and equine encephalitis. Note that two of these targets are toxins (botulinum and ricin) while the remainder are infectious agents.

Role of Public Health Departments and Disease Surveillance

It is important to note that all of the classical and modern biological weapons organisms are animal diseases, the only exception being smallpox. Thus, in any use of biological weapons, it is highly likely that animals will become ill either simultaneously with, or perhaps earlier than humans.

Indeed, in the largest biological weapons accident known– the anthrax outbreak in Sverdlovsk (now Yekaterinburg) in the Soviet Union in 1979, sheep became ill with anthrax as far as 200 kilometres from the release point of the organism from a military facility in the southeastern portion of the city. Thus, a robust surveillance system involving human clinicians and veterinarians may identify a bioweapons attack early in the course of an epidemic, permitting the prophylaxis of disease in the vast majority of people (and/or animals) exposed but not yet ill.

For example in the case of anthrax, it is likely that by 24 – 36 hours after an attack, some small percentage of individuals (those with compromised immune system or who had received a large dose of the organism due to proximity to the release point) will become ill with classical symptoms and signs (including a virtually unique chest X-ray finding, often recognized by public health officials if they receive timely reports). By making these data available to local public health officials in real time, most models of anthrax epidemics indicate that more than 80% of an exposed population can receive antibiotic treatment before becoming symptomatic, and thus avoid the moderately high mortality of the disease.

Identification of Bioweapons

The goal of biodefence is to integrate the sustained efforts of the national and homeland security, medical, public health, intelligence, diplomatic, and law enforcement communities. Health care providers and public health officers are among the first lines of defence. In some countries private, local, and provincial (state) capabilities are being augmented by and coordinated with federal assets, to provide layered defences against biological weapons attacks. During the first Gulf War the United Nations activated a biological and chemical response team, Task Force Scorpio, to respond to any potential use of weapons of mass destruction on civilians.

The traditional approach toward protecting agriculture, food, and water: focusing on the natural or unintentional introduction of a disease is being strengthened by focused efforts to address current and anticipated future biological weapons threats that may be deliberate, multiple, and repetitive. The growing threat of biowarfare agents and bioterrorism has led to the development of specific field tools that perform on-the-spot analysis and identification of encountered suspect materials. One such technology, being developed by researchers from the Lawrence Livermore National Laboratory (LLNL), employs a "sandwich immunoassay", in which fluorescent dye-labelled antibodies aimed at specific pathogens are attached to silver and gold nanowires.

In the Netherlands, the company TNO has designed Bioaerosol Single Particle Recognition eQuipment (BiosparQ). This system would be implemented into the national response plan for bioweapons attacks in the Netherlands.

Researchers at Ben Gurion University in Israel are developing a different device called the BioPen, essentially a "Lab-in-a-Pen", which can detect known biological agents in under 20 minutes using an adaptation of the ELISA, a similar widely employed immunological technique, that in this case incorporates fibre optics.

History

Biological warfare has been practiced repeatedly throughout history. Before the 20th century, the use of biological agents took three major forms:

- Deliberate poisoning of food and water with infectious material
- Use of microorganisms, toxins or animals, living or dead, in a weapon system
- Use of biologically inoculated fabrics.

Antiquity

The earliest documented incident of the intention to use biological weapons is recorded in Hittite texts of 1500–1200 B.C, in which victims of plague were driven into enemy lands. Although the Assyrians knew of ergot, a parasitic fungus of rye which produces ergotism when ingested, there is no evidence that they poisoned enemy wells with the fungus, as has been claimed.

According to Homer's epic poems about the legendary Trojan War, the *Iliad* and the *Odyssey,* spears and arrows were tipped with poison. During the First Sacred War in Greece, in about 590 BC, Athens and the Amphictionic League poisoned the water supply of the besieged town of Kirrha (near Delphi) with the toxic plant hellebore. The Roman commander Manius Aquillus poisoned the wells of besieged enemy cities in about 130 BC.

During the 4th century BC Scythian archers tipped their arrow tips with snake venom, human blood, and animal feces to cause wounds to become infected. There are numerous other instances of the use of plant toxins, venoms, and other poisonous substances to create biological weapons in antiquity.

In 184 B.C, Hannibal of Carthage had clay pots filled with venomous snakes and instructed his soldiers to throw the pots onto the decks of Pergamene ships. In about AD 198, the Parthian city of Hatra (near Mosul, Iraq) repulsed the Roman army led by Septimius Severus by hurling clay pots filled with live scorpions at them.

Middle Ages

The Mongol Empire established commercial and political connections between the Eastern and Western areas of the world, but it did so through the most mobile army ever seen. The armies, being the most rapidly moving travelers who had ever moved between the steppes of East Asia (where bubonic plague was and remains endemic among small rodents) and managed to keep the chain of infection without a break until they reached, and infected, peoples and rodents who had never encountered it. The ensuing Black Death may have killed almost half of the population of Europe in the next decades, changing the course of Asian and European history.

During the Middle Ages, victims of the bubonic plague were used for biological attacks, often by flinging the infected corpses (formites)and excrement over castle walls using catapults. In 1346, during the siege of Kafa (now Feodossia Ukraine) the attacking Tartar Forces which were subjugated by the Mongol empire under Genghis Khan, used the bodies of Mongol warriors of the Golden Horde who had died of plague, as weapons. The dead warriors were thrown over the walls of the besieged city of Crimean. An outbreak of plague followed and the defending forces retreated, followed by the conquest of the city by the Mongol army. It has been speculated that this operation may have been responsible for the advent of the Black Death in Europe.

At the siege of Thun-l'Eveque in 1340, during the Hundred Years' War, the attackers catapulted decomposing animals into the besieged area. In 1422, during the siege of Karlstein Castle in Bohemia, Hussite attackers used catapults to throw dead (but not plague-infected) bodies and 2000 carriage-loads of dung over the walls. The last known incident of using plague corpses for biological warfare occurred in 1710, when Russian forces attacked the Swedes by flinging plague-infected corpses over the city walls of Reval (Tallinn). However, during the 1785 siege of La Calle, Tunisian forces flung diseased clothing into the city.

18th Century

The Native American population was devastated after contact with the Old World due to the introduction of many different fatal diseases. There are two documented cases of alleged and attempted germ warfare. The first, during a parley at Fort Pitt on June 24, 1763, Ecuyer gave representatives of the besieging Delawares two blankets and a handkerchief that had been exposed to smallpox, hoping to spread the disease to the Natives in order to end the siege. William Trent, the militia commander, left records that clearly indicated that the purpose of giving the blankets was "to Convey the Smallpox to the Indians."

British commander Lord Jeffrey Amherst and Swiss-British officer Colonel Henry Bouquet certainly discussed this, in the course of Pontiac's Rebellion; there still exists correspondence referencing the idea of giving smallpox-infected blankets to enemy Indians. Historian Francis Parkman verifies four letters from June 29, July 13, 16 and 26th, 1763. Excerpts: Commander Lord Jeffrey Amherst writes July 16, 1763, "P.S. You will Do well to try to Inocculate the Indians by means of Blankets, as well as to try Every other method that can serve to Extirpate this Execrable Race. I should be very glad your Scheme for Hunting them Down by Dogs could take Effect,..." Colonel Henry Bouquet replies July 26, 1763, "I received yesterday your Excellency's letters of 16th with their Inclosures. The signal for Indian Messengers, and all your directions will be observed."

While the intent of carrying out biological warfare is clear, there is debate among historians as to whether this actually took place despite Bouquet's affirmative reply to Amherst, and the continuing correspondence on the point. Smallpox is highly infectious and does not require contaminated blankets to spread uncontrollably, and together with measles, influenza, chicken pox, etc. had been doing so since the arrival of Europeans and their animals. Historians have been unable to establish whether or not the Amherst plan was implemented, particularly in light of the fact that smallpox was already present in the region, and that scientific knowledge of disease at that time had yet to develop an understanding of infection vectors, nor in the case of smallpox a full acknowledgment of the protective effect of a cowpox infection.

Regardless of whether the plan was carried out, trade and combat provided ample opportunity for transmission of the disease. The diseases which depopulated the New World can be traced to Eurasia where people had long lived with them and developed some immunological ability to survive their presence. Without similarly long ancestral exposure, indigenous Americans were immunologically naive and extremely vulnerable.

19th Century

In 1834, Massachusetts diarist Richard Henry Dana visited San Francisco on a merchant ship. His ship traded many items including blankets with Mexicans and Russians who had established outposts on the northern side of the San Francisco Bay. Local histories document that the California plague epidemic began at the Russian fort soon after they left. It is possible that the blankets were the source of the contamination (hidden fleas, or rats, perhaps), but another possible source was a Chinese ship making port in San Francisco at the same time. Plague became established in California and has since become endemic throughout much of the North American West. Native rodents have suffered a severe population decline, only partly due to human eradication action.

During the American Civil War, General Sherman reported that Confederate forces shot farm animals in ponds upon which the Union troops depended for drinking water. This would have made the water unpleasant to drink, though perhaps the death caused might not have been that desired. A Confederate doctor planned and may have carried out a bacteriological attack on Northern populations across the Canadian border.

Jack London, in his story "'Yah! Yah! Yah!'", described a punitive European expedition to a South Pacific island deliberately exposing the Polynesian population to measles, of which many of them died. While much of the material for London's *South Sea Tales* is derived from his personal experience in the region, it is not known whether this particular incident is historical.

20th Century

During the First World War, the Empire of Germany pursued an ambitious biological warfare program. Using diplomatic pouches and couriers, the German General Staff supplied small teams of saboteurs in the Russian Duchy of Finland, and in the then-neutral countries of Romania, the United States, and Argentina.

In Finland, saboteurs mounted on reindeer placed ampoules of anthrax in stables of Russian horses in 1916. Anthrax was also supplied to the German military attache in Bucharest, as was glanders, which was employed against livestock destined for Allied service.

German intelligence officer and US citizen Dr. Anton Casimir Dilger established a secret lab in the basement of his sister's home in Chevy Chase, Maryland, that produced glanders which was used to infect livestock in ports and inland collection points including, at least, Newport News, Norfolk, Baltimore, and New York, and probably St. Louis and Covington, Kentucky. In Argentina, German agents also employed glanders in the port of Buenos Aires and also tried to ruin wheat harvests with a destructive fungus.

The Geneva Protocol of 1925 prohibited the use of chemical weapons and biological weapons, but said nothing about experimentation, production, storage, or transfer; later treaties did cover these aspects. Twentieth-century advances in microbiology enabled the first pure-culture biological agents to be developed by World War II.

The interwar period was a period of development by many nations, most notably the Empire of Japan. Secret Imperial Japanese Army Unit 731, based primarily at Pingfan in Manchuria commanded by Lieutenant General Shirô Ishii, did research on BW, conducted often fatal human experiments on prisoners, and produced biological weapons for combat use during the Second Sino-Japanese War.

Biological experiments, often using twins with one subject to the procedure and the other as a control, were carried out by Nazi Germany on concentration camp inmates, particularly by Joseph Mengele.

1937–1945

During the Sino-Japanese War (1937–1945) and World War II, the Imperial Japanese Army made use of biological weapons against both Chinese soldiers and civilians in several military campaigns. Three veterans of Unit 731 testified, in a 1989 interview to the Asahi Shimbun, that they were part of a mission to contaminate the Horustein river with typhoid near the Soviet troops during the Battle of Khalkhin Gol. In 1940, the Imperial Japanese Army Air Force bombed Ningbo with ceramic bombs full of fleas carrying the bubonic plague. A film showing this operation was seen by the imperial princes Tsuneyoshi Takeda and Takahito Mikasa during a screening made by mastermind Shiro Ishii. During the Khabarovsk War Crime Trials the accused, such as Major General Kiyashi Kawashima, testified that as early as 1941 some 40 members of Unit 731 air-dropped plague-contaminated fleas on Changde. These operations caused epidemic plague outbreaks.

Many operations were ineffective due to inefficient delivery systems, using disease-bearing insects rather than dispersing the agent as an bioaerosol cloud. Nevertheless, some modern Chinese historians estimate that 400,000 Chinese died as a direct result of Japanese field testing and operational use of biological weapons. In response to biological weapons development in Japan, and at the time suspected in Nazi Germany, the United States, United Kingdom, and Canada initiated a BW development programs in 1941 that resulted in the weaponization of tularemia, anthrax, brucellosis, and botulism toxin.

The centre for United States military BW research was Fort Detrick, Maryland, where USAMRIID is currently based; the first director was pharmaceutical executive George W. Merck. Some biological and chemical weapons research and testing was also conducted at Dugway Proving Grounds in Utah, at a munition manufacturing complex in Terre Haute, Indiana, and at a tract on Horn Island, Mississippi. Much of the British work was carried out at Porton Down. Field testing carried out in the United Kingdom during World War II left Gruinard island in Scotland contaminated with anthrax for the next 48 years.

1946 to 1972

During the 1948 Israel War of Independence, International Red Cross reports raised suspicion that the Jewish Haganah militia had released Salmonella typhi bacteria into the water supply for the city of Acre, causing an outbreak of typhoid among the inhabitants.

Egyptian troops later claimed to have captured disguised Haganah soldiers near wells in Gaza, whom they executed for allegedly attempting another attack. Israel denies these allegations.

During the Cold War, US conscientious objectors were used as consenting test subjects for biological agents in a program known as Operation Whitecoat. There were also many unpublicized tests carried out on the public during the Cold War. Considerable research on the topic was performed by the United States, the Soviet Union, and probably other major nations throughout the Cold War era, though it is generally believed that biological weapons were never used after World War II. This view was challenged by China and North Korea, who accused the United States of germ warfare in the Korean War (1950–1953).

Cuba has also accused the United States of spreading human and animal disease on their island nation. At the time of the Korean War the United States had only weaponized one agent, brucellosis ("Agent US"), which is caused by *Brucella suis*. The original weaponized form used the M114 bursting bomblet in M33 cluster bombs.

While the specific form of the biological bomb was classified until some years after the Korean War, in the various exhibits of biological weapons that Korea alleged were dropped on their country nothing resembled an M114 bomblet. There were ceramic containers that had some similarity to Japanese weapons used against the Chinese in World War II, developed by Unit 731.

Some of the Unit 731 personnel were imprisoned by the Soviets, and would have been a potential source of information on Japanese weaponization. The head of Unit 731, Lieutenant General Shiro Ishii, was granted immunity from war crimes prosecution in exchange for providing information to the United States on the Unit's activities.

The Korean War allegations also stressed the use of disease vectors, such as fleas, which, again, were probably a legacy of Japanese biological warfare efforts. The United States initiated its weaponization efforts with disease vectors in 1953, focused on Plague-fleas, EEE-mosquitoes, and yellow fever- mosquitoes (OJ-AP). However, US medical scientists in occupied Japan undertook extensive research on insect vectors, with the assistance of former Unit 731 staff, as early as 1946.

The United States Air Force was not satisfied with the operational qualities of the M114/US and labelled it an interim item until the United States Army Chemical Corps could deliver a superior weapon.

The Air Force also changed its plans and wanted lethal biologicals. The Chemical Corps then initiated a crash program to weaponize anthrax (N) in the E61 1/2-lb hour-glass bomblet. Though the program was successful in meeting its development goals, the lack of validation on the infectivity of anthrax stalled standardization.

Around 1950 the Chemical Corps also initiated a program to weaponize tularemia (UL). Shortly after the E61/N failed to make standardization, tularemia was standardized in the 3.4" M143 bursting spherical bomblet. This was intended for delivery by the MGM-29 Sergeant missile warhead and could produce 50% infection over a 7-square-mile (18 km^2) area. Unlike anthrax, tularemia had a demonstrated infectivity with human volunteers (Operation Whitecoat). Furthermore, although tularemia is treatable by antibiotics, treatment does not shorten the course of the disease.

In addition to the use of bursting bomblets for creating biological aerosols, the Chemical Corps started investigating aerosol-generating bomblets in the 1950s. The E99 was the first workable design, but was too complex to be manufactured. By the late 1950s the 4.5" E120 spraying spherical bomblet was developed; a B-47 bomber with a SUU-24/A dispenser could infect 50% or more of the population of a 16-square-mile (41 km^2) area with tularemia with the E120. The E120 was later superseded by dry-type agents.

Dry-type biologicals resemble talcum powder, and can be disseminated as aerosols using gas expulsion devices instead of a burster or complex sprayer. The Chemical Corps developed Flettner rotor bomblets and later triangular bomblets for wider coverage due to improved glide angles over Magnus-lift spherical bomblets. Weapons of this type were in advanced development by the time the program ended.

United States President Richard Nixon signed an executive order on November 1969, which stopped production of biological weapons in the United States and allowed only scientific research of lethal biological agents and defensive measures such as immunization and biosafety. The biological munition stockpiles were destroyed, and approximately 2,200 researchers became redundant.

United States Special Forces and the CIA also had an interest in biological warfare, and a series of special munitions was created for their operations. The covert weapons developed for the military (M1, M2, M4, M5, and M32- or Big Five Weapons) were destroyed in accordance with Nixon's executive order to end the offensive program.

The CIA maintained its collection of biologicals well into 1975 when it became the subject of the senate Church Committee.

The Biological Weapons Convention

In 1972, the United States signed the Biological and Toxic Weapons Convention, which banned the "development, production and stockpiling of microbes or their poisonous products except in amounts necessary for protective and peaceful research." By 1996, 137 countries had signed the treaty; however it is believed that since the signing of the Convention the number of countries capable of producing such weapons has increased.

The Soviet Union continued research and production of offensive biological weapons in a program called Biopreparat, despite having signed the convention. The United States was unaware of the program until Dr. Vladimir Pasechnik defected in 1989, and Dr. Kanatjan Alibekov, the first deputy director of Biopreparat defected in 1992.

After the 1991 Persian Gulf War, Iraq admitted to the United Nations inspection team to having produced 19,000 litres of concentrated botulinum toxin, of which approximately 10,000 L were loaded into military weapons; the 19,000 litres have never been fully accounted for. This is approximately three times the amount needed to kill the entire current human population by inhalation, although in practice it would be impossible to distribute it so efficiently, and, unless it is protected from oxygen, it deteriorates in storage.

On September 18, 2001 and for a few days after several letters were received by members of the United States Congress and media outlets containing anthrax spores: the attack killed five people. The identity of the perpetrator remained unknown until 2008, when a primary suspect was named.

Bibliography

Awasthi, A.K. : *A Textbook of Immunology*, Wisdom Press, Delhi, 2023.

Bandyopadhyay, P C : *Breeding and Crop Production*, Gene Tech Books, Delhi, 2017.

Bhagwan, Pooja : *A Handbook of Inorganic Chemistry : Nuclear, Atomic, Aqueous, Alkali and Alkaline*, ISPA, Delhi, 2015.

Chaudhary, Vikas : *Entomology and Pest Management*, Navyug, Delhi, 2018.

Cristobal Noe Aguilar : *Food Science and Food Biotechnology in Developing Countries*, Asiatech Pub, 2018.

Dharamvir Hota: *Modern Biotechnology in Plant Breeding*, Gene Tech Books, Delhi, 2017.

Dodia, DA ; IS Patel and GM Patel: *Botanical Pesticides for Pest Management*, Scientific, Delhi, 2019.

Garg, G.P. : *Medicinal Biochemistry*, Discovery Publishing House, Delhi, 2023.

Gilbert Wooding Robinson: *Soils : Their Origin Constitution and Classification*, Biotech Books, Delhi, 2015.

Hota, Dharamvir : *Modern Biotechnology in Plant Breeding*, Gene Tech Books, Delhi, 2017.

Iqbal, S.A. and M. Satake: *An Introduction to Analytical Chemistry*, Discovery, Delhi, 2009.

Jain, Sumit: *Biotech's Dictionary of Plant Breeding and Genetics*, Biotech, Delhi, 2015.

Jawaid A. Khan and Jeanne Dijkstra : *Handbook of Plant Virology*, Heritage Pub, 2017.

Keshav Prasad Yadav: *Application of Morphometry in Geomorphology*, Radha Pub, Delhi, 2018.

Khan, Samiullah : *Plant Breeding Advances and in vitro Culture*, CBS, Delhi, 2007.

Leena Parihar: *Dairy Microbiology*, Agrobios, Delhi, 2018.

Matsuoka H.: *Cultivation of Panicum Genetic Resources for Evaluation of Characteristics*, Tokyo, JICA, 2017.

Mishra, Shubhrata R. : *Morphology of Fungi*, Discovery Pub, Delhi, 2015.

Narang, R.K.: *Fruit and Vegetable Preservation Techniques*, APH Pub, Delhi, 2020.

Panjarathinam, R. : *A Textbook of Medical Parasitology*, Universities Press, Delhi, 2017.

Pareek O. P.: *Advances in Horticulture: Fruit Crops,* New Delhi, Malhotra Publishing House, 2019.

Raghunath Narvekar: *Handbook of Biochemistry*, Adhyayan, Delhi, 2018.

Ramann, E. : *The Evolution and Classification of Soils*, Asiatic Pub, Calcutta, 2016.

Shalini, S.: *Vedic Leguminous Plants (Medicinal and Microbiological Study)*, Classical, Delhi, 2007.

Sharma, R.C. : *Diseases of Horticultural Crops: Fruits*, Indus, Delhi, 2019.

Tyagi, Prasum : *A Textbook of Animal Physiology*, Dominant, Delhi, 2012.

Vanderplank, J.E.: *Plant Diseases: Epidemics and Control,* New York, NY, USA, Academic Press, 1993.

Vikas Chaudhary: *Entomology and Pest Management*, Navyug, Delhi, 2018.

William Alec : *The Chemical Industry*, London: Longman Group Limited, 2001.

Yoshida T.: *Cultivation of Citrus Genetic Resources for Evaluation of Characteristics*, Tokyo, JICA, 2006.

Index

❑❑❑